ADVANCES IN

Vascular Surgery®

VOLUME 7

ADVANCES IN

Vascular Surgery®

VOLUMES 1 THROUGH 4 (OUT OF PRINT)

VOLUME 5

Surgical Management of Recurrent Carotid Stenosis, *by William C. Mackey*

Endovascular Treatment of Brachiocephalic Lesions With Angioplasty and Stents, *by Edward B. Diethrich*

Brachiocephalic Arterial Revascularization: A Surgical Perspective, *by John W. Hallett, Jr.*

Diagnosis and Treatment of Upper Extremity Ischemia, *by W. Kent Williamson, Mark R. Nehler, Lloyd M. Taylor, Jr., and John M. Porter*

Failing and Failed Hemodialysis Access Sites, *by Jeffrey L. Kaufman*

Critical Pathways for Abdominal Aortic Aneurysms, *by Keith D. Calligaro, Rahul Dandura, Matthew J. Dougherty, Carol A. Raviola, and Dominic A. DeLaurentis*

Epidural Cooling for the Prevention of Spinal Cord Ischemic Complications After Thoracoabdominal Aortic Surgery, *by Richard P. Cambria and J. Kenneth Davison*

Utility of Spiral CT in the Preoperative Evaluation of Patients with Abdominal Aortic Aneurysms, *by Mark F. Fillinger*

Laparoscopic Aortic Surgery, *by Carlos R. Gracia and Yves-Marie Dion*

Management of Mycotic Aneurysms, *by Dennis F. Bandyk*

Directional Atherectomy: Indications, Devices, Techniques, and Results, *by Stephen T. Kee, Charles P. Semba, and Michael D. Dake*

The Natural History of Renal Artery Disease, *by R. Eugene Zierler*

Options for Anticoagulation, *by Timothy K. Liem and Donald Silver*

The Role of Growth Factors in Lower Extremity Ischemia and Nonhealing Wounds, *by Robert Y. Rhee, Marshall W. Webster, and David L. Steed*

VOLUME 6

Impact of Plaque Morphology in Carotid Disease, *by Nancy L. Cantelmo*

Management of Complications of Aortic Dissection, *by David C. Brewster*

Treatment of Infected Aortic Grafts With In Situ Aortic Reconstruction Using Superficial Femoral-Popliteal Veins, *by Ryan T. Hagino and G. Patrick Clagett*

Update Regarding Current Utility of Endoluminal Prostheses for Aortoiliac Disease, *by Michael L. Marin, Larry H. Hollier, Harold A. Mitty, Richard Parsons, and James M. Cooper*

Endoleak—A Complication Unique to Endovascular Grafting: The Sydney Experience, *by James May and Geoffrey H. White*

Evolution of Varicose Vein Surgery, *by John J. Bergan*

Balloon Dissection for Endoscopic Subfascial Ligation, *by Roy L. Tawes, L. Albert Wetter, Gerald R. Sydorak, George D. Hermann, and Thomas J. Fogarty*

Renal Revascularization for Salvage: Results of Treatment for Renal Artery Occlusion, *by Kimberley J. Hansen and Timothy C. Oskin*

Current Management of the Ischemic Hand, *by Christian E. Sampson, and Julian J. Pribaz*

Role of Dublex Imaging Before Infrainguinal Bypass, *by D.E. Standness, Jr.*

Role of Magnetic Resonance Angiography in Peripheral Vascular Disease, *by William D. Turnipseed and Thomas M. Grist*

Endoscopic Techniques for Harvesting the Greater Saphenous Vein, *by Jae-Sung Cho and Peter Gloviczki*

Management of the Thrombosed Infrainguinal Vein Graft, *by Daniel B. Walsh*

Subintimal (Extraluminal) Angioplasty of Femoropopliteal, Iliac, and Tibial Vessels, *by Amman Bolia and Peter Bell*

Creative Foot Salvage, *by John E. Connolly, Martha D. McDaniel, James S. Wrobel, and Kim M. Rozokat*

Gene Therapy for Vascular Disease, *by Michael J. Mann and Michael S. Conte*

ADVANCES IN

Vascular Surgery®

VOLUME 7

Editor-in-Chief
Anthony D. Whittemore, M.D.
Chief Medical Officer, Chief, Division of Vascular Surgery, Brigham and Women's Hospital; Professor of Surgery, Harvard Medical School, Boston, MA

Associate Editors
Dennis F. Bandyk, M.D.
Professor of Surgery, University of South Florida College of Medicine; Director, Vascular Surgery Division, Tampa, Florida

Jack L. Cronenwett, M.D.
Professor of Surgery, Dartmough Medical School; Chief, Section of Vascular Surgery, Dartmouth–Hitchcock Medical Center, Lebanon, New Hampshire

Norman Hertzer, M.D.
Department of Vascular Surgery, Cleveland Clinic Foundation, Cleveland, Ohio

Rodney A. White, M.D.
Professor of Surgery, University of California at Los Angeles School of Medicine; Chief of Vascular Surgery, Associate Chairman, Department of Surgery, Harbor–University of California at Los Angeles Medical Center, Torrance, California

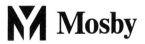 Mosby

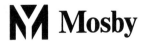 **Mosby**

Publisher: Theresa Van Schaik
Developmental Editor: Sarah A. Zagarri
Manager, Periodical Editing: Kirk Swearingen
Production Editor: Amanda Maguire
Project Supervisor, Production: Joy Moore
Production Assistant: Karie House

Printed in the United States of America
Printing/binding by The Maple-Vail Book Manufacturing Group

Editorial Office:
Mosby, Inc.
11830 Westline Industrial Drive
St. Louis, MO 63146
Customer Service: customer.support@mosby.com

www.mosby.com/Mosby/CustomerSupport/index.html

International Standard Serial Number: 1069-7292
International Standard Book Number: 0-8151-8416-6

Contributors

Joseph Patrick Archie, Jr., M.D., Ph.D.
Clinical Professor of Surgery, University of North Carolina, Chapel Hill,
North Carolina; Adjunct Professor of Mechanical and Aerospace
Engineering, North Carolina State University, Raleigh, North Carolina

Jan D. Blankensteijn, M.D.
Professor of Vascular Surgery, University of Utrecht; Consultant Vascular
Surgeon, Department of Vascular Surgery, University Hospital Utrecht,
Utrecht, The Netherlands

Christina M. Braun, R.N.
Vascular Nurse Clinician, The Miriam Hospital, Providence, Rhode
Island

David P. Brophy, M.D.
Assistant Professor of Radiology, Harvard Medical School, Boston,
Massachusetts; Cardiovascular and Interventional Radiologist,
Department of Radiology, Beth Israel Deaconess Medical Center, Boston
Massachusetts

Joaquim J. Cerveira, M.D.
Vascular Fellow, Division of Vascular Surgery, Long Island Jewish
Medical Center, New Hyde Park, New York

Benjamin B. Chang, M.D.
Assistant Professor of Surgery, Albany Medical College, Surgeon, Albany
Medical Center, Albany, New York

Jon R. Cohen, M.D.
Professor of Surgery, Albert Einstein School of Medicine, Bronx, New
York; Chairman, Department of Surgery, Long Island Jewish Medical
Center, New Hyde Park, New York

Andrea M. Colucci, R.N.
Vascular Nurse Clinician, The Miriam Hospital, Providence, Rhode
Island

R. Clement Darling III, M.D.
Associate Professor of Surgery, Albany Medical College, Chief, Division
of Vascular Surgery, Albany Medical Center, Albany, New York

Bert C. Eikelboom, M.D.
Associate Professor of Vascular Surgery, University of Utrecht; Chief,
Department of Vascular Surgery, University Hospital Utrecht, Utrecht,
The Netherlands

James M. Estes, M.D.
Assistant Professor of Surgery, Tufts University School of Medicine, Staff Surgeon, New England Medical Center, Boston, Massachusetts

Brian L. Ferris, M.D.
Resident, Vascular Surgery, Division of Vascular Surgery, Department of Surgery, Oregon Health Sciences University, Protland, Oregon

E. John Harris, Jr., M.D.
Assistant Professor of Surgery, Division of Vascular Surgery, Stanford University School of Medicine, Stanford, California; Medical Director, Stanford Vascular Laboratory

Paul B. Kreienberg, M.D.
Assistant Professor of Surgery, Albany Medical College, Surgeon, Albany Medical Center, Albany, New York

William E. Lloyd, M.D.
Assistant Professor of Surgery, Albany Medical College, Surgeon, Albany Medical Center, Albany, New York

Gregory L. Moneta, M.D.
Professor of Surgery, Division of Vascular Surgery, Department of Surgery, Oregon Health Sciences University, Portland, Oregon; Department of Veterans Affairs Hospital, Portland, Oregon

Robert B. Patterson, M.D.
Associate Professor of Surgery, Associate Surgeon-in-Chief; Chief, Peripheral Vascular Surgery; Medical Director, Vascular Exercise Program; Co-director, Noninvasive Vascular Laboratory, Department of Surgery, Division of Vascular Surgery, Brown University School of Medicine, Providence, Rhode Island; The Miriam Hospital, Providence, Rhode Island

Philip S.K. Paty, M.D.
Associate Professor of Surgery, Albany Medical College, Surgeon, Albany Medical Center, Albany, New York

Laura J. Perry, M.D.
Instructor of Radiology, Harvard Medical School, Boston, Massachusetts; Angiographer and Interventional Radiologist, Department of Radiology, Beth Israel Deaconess Medical Center, Boston, Massachusetts

David B. Pilcher, M.D.
Professor of Surgery, Division of Vascular and Transplant Surgery, Department of Surgery, University of Vermont College of Medicine, Burlington, Vermont

Michael A. Ricci, M.D.
Associate Professor of Surgery, Division of Vascular and Transplant Surgery, Department of Surgery, University of Vermont College of Medicine, Burlington, Vermont

David Rosenthal, M.D.
Clinical Professor of Surgery, Medical College of Georgia, Georgia Baptist
Medical Center, Atlanta, Georgia

Brian G. Rubin, M.D.
Assistant Professor of Surgery, Division of General Surgery, Section of
Vascular Surgery, Washington University School of Medicine, Barnes-
Jewish Hospital, St. Louis, Missouri

Timur P. Sarac, M.D.
Vascular Surgery Fellow, University of Florida College of Medicine,
Division of Vascular Surgery, Gainesville, Florida

James M. Seeger, M.D.
Professor and Chief of Vascular Surgery, University of Florida College of
Medicine, Division of Vascular Surgery, Gainesville, Florida

Dhiraj M. Shah, M.D.
Professor of Surgery, Albany Medical College, Director, Vascular
Institute, Albany Medical Center, Albany, New York

Gregorio A. Sicard, M.D.
Professor of Surgery and Radiology, Washington University School of
Medicine, Chief, Division of General Surgery and Section of Vascular
Surgery, Barnes-Jewish Hospital, St. Louis, Missouri

Robert B. Smith III, M.D.
John E. Skandalakis Professor of Surgery, Division of Vascular Surgery,
Emory University School of Medicine, Atlanta, Georgia; Medical
Director, Emory University Hospital, Atlanta, Georgia

Thomas W. Wakefield, M.D.
Professor of Surgery, Section of Vascular Surgery, Department of Surgery,
University of Michigan, Ann Arbor, Michigan

Victor J. Weiss, M.D.
Fellow in Vascular Surgery, Division of Vascular Surgery, Emory
University School of Medicine, Atlanta, Georgia

Contents

Contributors   ix

PART I Carotid Artery Disease

1. **Carotid Endarterectomy Outcomes: Trials, Regional and Statewide Studies, Individual Surgeon Variance, and the Influence of Patch Reconstruction and Patch Materials**
   By Joseph Patrick Archie, Jr.   1

   Perioperative Stroke and/or Stroke and Death Rates for Prospective, Randomized Trials, Regional and Statewide Studies, and Pooled Data Reports   3

   Individual Surgeon Outcome Variance and Computational Methods   6

   Prospective Randomized Trials Comparing Primary Closure With Patch Angioplasty Reconstruction   8

   Outcomes of Prospective Randomized and Nonrandomized Studies Comparing Patching With Primary Closure   10

   Practical and Theoretical Advantages of Patch Reconstruction Over Primary Closure   13

   Effect of Patch Material on Outcomes   14

   Conclusion   18

2. **Decision Making for Asymptomatic Patients With Critical Carotid Stenosis**
   By James M. Estes   23

   Impact of Prospective Randomized Trials   23

   Impact of Demographics and Co-morbidity   24

   Characteristics of Patient Sample   26

   Perioperative Morbidity and Mortality   26

   Long-term Follow-up   28

   Conclusions   30

Carotid Endarterectomy Outcome and Cardiac
Disease   30

Carotid Endarterectomy Outcome and Other
Co-morbidities   31

Carotid Endarterectomy Outcome and Age   31

Comments   32

Clinical Relevance   33

Age and Co-morbidity   33

Hospital and Surgeon Case Volume   34

Future Prospects   36

**3. Duplex Scanning and Spectral Analysis of Carotid
Artery Occlusive Disease: Improving Relevance to
Clinical Practice**
By Brian L. Ferris and Gregory L. Moneta   41

Quantification of ICA Stenosis   42

Supplemental Duplex Criteria   46

Nascet Duplex Criteria   47

ACAS Duplex Criteria   49

Bilateral ICA Stenosis   50

4. Carotid Endarterectomy by the Eversion Technique
*By Dhiraj M. Shah, R. Clement Darling III, Benjamin B.
Chang, Paul B. Kreienberg, Philip S.K. Paty, and
William E. Lloyd*   55

Methods   58

Selection of Cases   58

Perioperative Management   59

Technique   60

Use of a Shunt   68

Nonredundant Carotids   70

Technical Suggestions   70

Clinical Materials and Results   71

Conclusion   74

5. Management of Carotid Kinks and Coils
By Victor J. Weiss and Robert B. Smith III   77
  Incidence   77
  Etiology   78
  Signs and Symptoms   78
  Diagnosis   79
  Indications for Surgery   79
  Surgical Management   80
  Conclusion   83

PART II Aortic Disease

6. Endovascular Treatment of Abdominal Aortic Aneurysms
By Gregorio A. Sicard and Brian G. Rubin   87
  Historical Perspective   88
  Characteristics of Endovascular AAA Grafts   89
    Attachment Systems   89
    Graft Support Systems   92
    Graft Material   92
    Modular Versus Single-Unit Design   92
    Delivery Systems   93
    Deployment Systems   94
  Selection of Patients for Endovascular AAA Repair   94
  Results of Endovascular AAA Repair   96
    Technical Success and Mortality   96
  Complications   96
  Summary   103

7. How and When to Treat an Endoleak After Endovascular Abdominal Aortic Aneurysm Repair
By Bert C. Eikelboom and Jan D. Blankensteijn   105
  Endoleaks   106
  Consequences of an Endoleak   107

The Unpredictability of Endoleaks   107

Case Descriptions   109

    Case 1   109

    Case 2   112

    Case 3   113

    Case 4   115

What is Known About Treating Endoleaks?   116

Follow-up Imaging   118

Our Approach to the Endoleak Problem   119

Conclusion   120

8. Laparoscopic Surgery for Abdominal Aortic Aneurysms

By Joaquim J. Cerveira and Jon R. Cohen   123

    Use of Laparoscopy in Vascular Surgery   124

    Operative Technique   125

    Clinical Experience   128

        Lessons Learned   132

    Future Developments   133

    Conclusion   134

PART III   Infrainguinal Disease

9. Endovascular In Situ Bypass

By David Rosenthal   137

    Technique of Operation   138

    Valvulotomy   138

    Side Branch Occlusion   139

10. The Current Role of a Supervised Exercise Program as Therapy for Arterial Claudication

By Robert B. Patterson, Andrea M. Colucci, and Christina M. Braun 147

    Components of the Brown Vascular Exercise Program 149

    Personnel and Equipment Requirements   149

    Space and Resources   149

Program Structure 150
  Phase 1 150
  Phase 2 153
  Phase 3 155
Results 155
  Patient Population 155
  Walking Ability 155
  Quality-of-Life Measurements 157
  Experience With Starting a Program 159
  Reimbursement 159
Discussion 160
  Natural History 160
  Drug Therapy 160
  Exercise Therapy 161
Conclusion 164

PART IV Anticoagulation

11. Anticoagulation for Infrainguinal Revascularization
By Timur P. Sarac and James M. Seeger 167
  Use of Anticoagulation to Improve Early Bypass Graft Patency 168
  Our Current Approach to Anticoagulation in the Immediate Postoperative Period 170
  Use of Anticoagulation to Improve Long-term Bypass Graft Patency 170
  Our Current Approach to Long-term Anticoagulation After an Infrainguinal Bypass 174
  Conclusion 176

12. Anticoagulants: Old and New
By Thomas W. Wakefield 179
  Basics of Coagulation 179
  Standard Unfractionated Heparin 181
    Low-Molecular Weight Heparin 183

Other Anticoagulants 185

  Hirudin 185

  Ancrod 185

  Antiplatelet Agents 186

PART V Imaging Techniques

13. Duplex Three-Dimensional Ultrasound: Potential Benefits

By E. John Harris, Jr. 189

  Development of Duplex US 190

  Development of a System 192

  Spatial Orientation 194

  Three-Dimensional Volume Visualization 195

  Preliminary Development at Stanford 196

  Potential Applications for Three-Dimensional US 197

PART VI Portal Hypertension

14. Transjugular Intrahepatic Portosystemic Shunts

By David P. Brophy and Laura J. Perry 199

  Indications and Contraindications 200

  Patient Preparation Before Transjugular Intrahepatic Portosystemic Shunting 204

  Procedural Technique 206

  Postprocedural Care 212

  Results 215

  Complications 215

  Transjugular Intrahepatic Portosystemic Shunting Patency and Surveillance 222

  Future 224

PART VII Basic Science

15. Pharmacologic Inhibition of Aortic Aneurysm Expansion

By Michael A. Ricci and David B. Pilcher 229

Beta-Blockade   230
  Experimental Evidence   230
  Clinical Evidence   232
Metalloproteinase Inhibition   235
  Indomethacin   236
  Doxycycline   236
Conclusion   237

Index   243

PART I

Carotid Artery Disease

CHAPTER 1

Carotid Endarterectomy Outcomes: Trials, Regional and Statewide Studies, Individual Surgeon Variance, and the Influence of Patch Reconstruction and Patch Materials

Joseph Patrick Archie, Jr., M.D., Ph.D.
Clinical Professor of Surgery, University of North Carolina, Chapel Hill, North Carolina; Adjunct Professor of Mechanical and Aerospace Engineering, North Carolina State University, Raleigh, North Carolina

Carotid endarterectomy (CEA) has been proven to be effective in stroke prevention for symptomatic patients with 50% diameter stenosis or greater[1,2] and for asymptomatic patients with 60% diameter stenosis or greater,[3] provided that they are properly selected and the operating surgeon has a combined 30-day perioperative stroke and death rate of less than 6% for symptomatic patients and less than 3% for asymptomatic patients. The degree of effectiveness of CEA is primarily determined by the minimization of perioperative morbidity and mortality. The lower a surgeon's perioperative stroke or death rate with respect to these thresholds of acceptability, the more effective stroke prevention is. Although the recommended upper threshold values of less than 6% and less than 3% are based on prospective randomized trials,[4-7] the mean values for perioperative outcomes in the respective trials are very close to these thresholds; therefore, the 95% confidence intervals (CIs) for the outcomes include the threshold values themselves.

Recent regional and statewide studies report perioperative CEA outcomes that are highly variable both between studies and within studies for hospitals and individual surgeons. This generates a number of concerns, including the general nationwide absence of monitoring of institutional and individual surgeon results and how to calculate them, the lack of a global acceptance and understanding of percent carotid diameter stenosis, the rapidly increasing rate of CEA for asymptomatic stenosis coupled with the difficulty of meeting the less than 3% threshold for perioperative stroke or death rates, and the perceived concept within the general medical community that all commonly applied CEA techniques produce similar results. Although the perioperative stroke or death rates for both symptomatic and asymptomatic patients appear to be independent of percent carotid stenosis,[1-3] it is not surprising that the stroke prevention value of CEA increases in each group in the presence of a higher percent of stenosis[2,8]

Given the current state of variability of CEA outcomes between regions, hospitals, and individual surgeons, it is important to address the issue of how best to achieve optimal outcomes. Provided that patients undergoing CEA fall within the guidelines set by the prospective randomized trials with respect to symptoms, risk factors, and percent stenosis, the major determinants of CEA outcomes are the decisions made by surgeons and the techniques they choose to use. If there are technical choices such as patching and patch material that may significantly improve outcomes, they need to be seriously considered, particularly by less experienced surgeons who do not have a clearly defined track record and by those with marginal or even unacceptable outcomes. The minimum 30-day perioperative stroke or death rate that can be achieved with CEA, or with any other interventional carotid procedure, is close to 1%. This figure is based on the known mortality rate from coronary artery disease in patients with carotid stenosis of approximately 0.5% per month and on the approximate 0.5% incidence of strokes caused by hyperperfusion syndrome after any form of carotid revascularization. The best perioperative stroke or death outcome of about 1% may decrease in the future with improved management of these problems. Although a reduction in the perioperative stroke or death rate from 6% for symptomatic patients or 3% for asymptomatic patients to the optimal figure of 1% seems small in absolute terms, the three- to fivefold level of outcome improvement clearly is significant from a clinical standpoint. As will be documented herein, highly frequent or obligatory reconstruction using patch angioplasty in general, and autologous greater saphenous vein patches specifically, is one way to achieve this gold standard.

This chapter reviews the currently published outcomes for CEA, identifies the correct way to compute individual surgeon outcomes, and presents data supporting CEA techniques that are beneficial in reducing the incidence of perioperative thrombosis and strokes as well as recurrent stenosis.

PERIOPERATIVE STROKE AND/OR STROKE AND DEATH RATES FOR PROSPECTIVE, RANDOMIZED TRIALS, REGIONAL AND STATEWIDE STUDIES, AND POOLED DATA REPORTS

The two most influential randomized trials comparing CEA to best medical management in the United States and Canada are the North American Symptomatic Carotid Endarterectomy Trial (NASCET)[1,2] and the Asymptomatic Carotid Atherosclerosis Study (ACAS).[3] A summary of the 30-day perioperative stroke and combined stroke or death rates for the two NASCET studies and the ACAS are given in Table 1. The two NASCET studies (70% diameter or greater stenosis and less than 70% diameter stenosis) have similar perioperative outcomes for both major strokes and minor ipsilateral strokes. A minor stroke was considered to be either nondisabling or completely resolved within 90 days after CEA. The pooled NASCET perioperative ipsilateral stroke rate was 6.0%, and the ipsilateral major stroke rate was 2.1%. The perioperative death rate was 0.5%. Of interest, the mean combined stroke or death rate (6.5%) for the pooled NASCET data exceeds the 6% maximum threshold value recommended for CEA in symptomatic patients.[4,5,7] The ACAS perioperative outcomes are more difficult to place into perspective because of the 1.2% incidence of strokes caused by diagnostic arteriography. In the first NASCET study, the stroke rate with arteriography was reported to be 0.7%, but this was not included in the outcome data because arteriography was performed before randomization. When only perioperative strokes are considered for the ACAS, the 1.5% incidence of perioperative strokes or death and the 95% CI are well below the 3% maximum threshold recommended for CEA in asymptomatic patients.[6,7] The perioperative stroke or death rates in these trials appear to be independent of percent carotid stenosis, but the potential benefit of CEA in stroke prevention increases with percent stenosis.[8] Although perioperative stroke rates may be independent of percent stenosis, they are higher in older patients, in females, and in patients with unstable neurologic status or crescendo transient ischemic attacks. However, the major determinant of a perioperative stroke is the surgeon.[9,10]

Recently published data on CEA perioperative outcomes from regional,[11] statewide,[12-15] multicenter,[16] and pooled reports[17,18]

TABLE 1.

Thirty-Day Perioperative Ipsilateral Stroke Rates for the Major Prospective Randomized Trials Comparing CEA With Medical Treatment

Study	Stroke		Stroke or Death	
	n	% (95% CI)	n	% (95% CI)
1. NASCET 1991[1] (70% to 99% stenosis)				
Major ipsilateral stroke	6/ 328	1.8% (0.4% to 3.2%)	7/ 328	2.1% (0.5% to 3.7%)
All ipsilateral strokes	18/ 328	5.5% (2.6% to 7.1%)	19/ 328	5.8% (3.3% to 8.3%)
2. NASCET 1998[2] (<70% stenosis)				
Major ipsilateral stroke	24/ 1,087	2.2% (1.3% to 3.1%)	30/ 1,087	3.0% (2.0% to 4.0%)
All ipsilateral strokes	67/ 1,087	6.2% (4.8% to 7.5%)	73/ 1,087	6.7% (5.3% to 8.3%)
3. ACAS 1995[3] (≥60% stenosis)				
Including arteriography	16/ 825	1.9% (1.0% to 2.8%)	19/ 825	2.3% (1.3% to 3.3%)
CEA only	7/ 721	1.0% (0.3% to 1.7%)	11/ 731	1.5% (0.6% to 2.4%)
4. Pooled NASCET 1991 and NASCET 1998[1,2]				
Major ipsilateral stroke	30/ 1,415	2.1% (1.4% to 2.8%)	37/ 1,415	2.6% (1.8% to 3.4%)
All ipsilateral strokes	85/ 1,415	6.0% (4.8% to 7.2%)	92/ 1,415	6.5% (5.2% to 7.8%)

Abbreviations: CEA, carotid endarterectomy; *CI*, confidence interval; *NASCET*, North American Symptomatic Carotid Endarterectomy Trial; *ACAS*, Asymptomatic Carotid Atherosclerosis Study.

are given in Table 2. The 4.5% perioperative stroke rate in the Toronto study[11] is similar to what would be expected from a mix of 73% symptomatic and 27% asymptomatic CEAs when compared with the pooled NASCET and ACAS data [6.0%(0.73) + 1.0%(0.27) = 4.6%]. The four statewide studies[12-15] have somewhat better outcomes but suffer from either incomplete participation or no external corroboration of reported results. For example, in the Maine study,[12] 362 CEAs were reported but another 258

TABLE 2.
Recent State, Regional, Multicenter, and Pooled Reports of Perioperative CEA Outcomes

Origin	Year Published	% Symptomatic/ % Asymptomatic	n	Stroke % (95% CI)	Stroke or Death % (95% CI)
1. Toronto[11]	1998	73%/27%	1,280	4.5% (3.4% to 5.6%)	6.3% (5.0% to 7.6%)
2. Maine[12]	1998	63%/37%	362	2.5% (0.9% to 4.1%)	2.8% (0.5% to 7.6%)
3. Maryland[13]	1998	N/A	9,918	0.9% (0.7% to 1.1%)	2.6% (2.3% to 2.9%)
4. Kentucky[14]	1997	57%/43%	986	1.0% (0.4% to 1.6%)	2.3% (1.4% to 3.2%)
5. Connecticut[15]	1996	N/A	3,833	N/A	4.7% (4.0% to 5.4%)
6. 12 Academic Centers[16]	1998	0%/100%	463	N/A	2.8% (1.3% to 4.3%)
7. 51 Pooled[17]	1996	100%/0%	15,956	N/A	5.6% (5.2% to 6.0%)
8. 25 Pooled[18]	1996	100%/0%	11,917	N/A	5.2% (4.8% to 5.6%)
9. 25 Pooled[18]	1996	0%/100%	3,139	N/A	3.4% (2.8% to 4.0%)

Abbreviations: CEA, carotid endarterectomy; *CI*, confidence interval; *N/A*, not applicable.

either were not reported (N = 153) or were done in nonparticipating hospitals (N = 105). There were four deaths in the latter two groups compared with only one death in the reported group (P = 0.10 by Fisher's exact test). Of the four statewide studies, the best outcomes came from an analysis of vascular surgeons' results.[14] The pooled data reports of combined perioperative stroke or death[17,18] rates for symptomatic and asymptomatic carotid stenosis are similar to those for the NASCET and the ACAS. However, excluding strokes related to preoperative arteriography, the perioperative stroke or death rate in the ACAS (1.5%) is significantly better than the 3.4% rate from pooled asymptomatic CEA data (P = 0.01 by chi-square analysis).[18]

INDIVIDUAL SURGEON OUTCOME VARIANCE AND COMPUTATIONAL METHODS

Several studies have demonstrated profound adverse outcomes when surgeons performed only a few operations per year: 1 or less CEA per year vs. more than 10 CEAs per year,[15] less than 6 CEAs per year vs. more than 12 CEAs per year,[11] and less than 5 CEAs per year vs. 5 or more CEAs per year.[19] In clinical practice, the outcomes of CEAs are determined by individual surgeons one operation at a time, not by hospitals per se, and depend on the competency of the surgeons who have privileges to perform CEAs. It is a leap of faith to conclude that any surgeon granted hospital privileges to perform CEAs can or will achieve acceptable results, much less gold standard results. Of equal concern is the frequent assumption by physicians who refer patients to any surgeon with privileges to perform CEAs that the outcome will be an acceptably low perioperative stroke rate. Unfortunately, referral patterns are complex and are influenced by multiple factors, not the least of which is who happens to contract with a provider with the low bid. Although the latter problem probably will be resolved, the overriding concerns of individual surgical expertise and outcome need to be addressed.

The marked variability of CEA outcomes among individual surgeons not only is disturbing but also is based on small numbers of operations in many instances.[15,19] Assessing one's own surgical outcomes can be both humbling and informative. If the number of procedures is N and the number of adverse events is n, the percent rate of events is easily calculated as $100n/N$. However, the 95% CI of the complication rate also is an extremely important number, especially when n and N are small. When the absolute number of events, n, is five or more, the $\pm$95% CI is routinely and correctly calculated from the normal distribution as $\pm 196[p(1 - p)/N]$,[12] where $p = n/N$. It is poorly understood and infrequently practiced that, when N is less than five, the binomial or Poisson distribution (a skewed distribution, not the normal distribution) must be used to determine the 95% CI. The values of this distribution are readily obtained from tables and graphs of this distribution when n and N are known. For example, if 100 CEAs have been performed ($N = 100$) and there were six strokes or deaths ($n = 6$; $n/N = p = 0.06$), the rate is 6.0% and the ±95% CI is ±196 $[0.06(0.94)/100]^{1/2} = ±4.6\%$. The 95% CI is 1.4% to 10.6% for strokes or death. If only three strokes or deaths occurred in 100 CEAs, the incorrect ±95% CI (because n is less than 5) from the normal distribution is $196[0.03(0.97)/100]^{1/2} = 3.3\%$, or −0.3% to 6.3%, which is impossible. Computed correctly from the binomial distribution for $N = 100$, $n = 3$, the 95% CI is 0% to 8.4%. It is clear that the mean rate of 3% may be satisfactory, but the 95% CI is too large.

Further problems with wide 95% CIs arise when the number of CEAs is small. For example, if 30 CEAs have been performed without a stroke or death ($n = 0$, $N = 30$), the 95% CI is 0% to 12% with a 35% chance that it is 6% or more. In other words, for the next CEA, there is a 95% probability that the chance of a stroke or death is less than 12%, but it clearly is not 0%. The only certain way to narrow the 95% CI is to have a large number of cases. This is well illustrated by the data provided in the tables throughout this chapter. This is a daunting problem that can only be resolved by a large experience with CEA.

Because adverse perioperative event rates for CEA, such as a stroke or death, usually are low, it is difficult for inexperienced or low-volume surgeons to get a firm idea about their outcomes. It has been suggested that one way to overcome this problem is to use 100 CEAs as a fixed minimum N value until the case load exceeds this number. Following this scenario for zero, one, two,..., six strokes or deaths, the 95% CIs are 0% to 4% for 0% strokes or death, 0% to 5.5% for 1%, 0% to 7% for 2%, 0.5% to 8.5% for 3%, 1.5% to 9.7% for 4%, 2% to 11.5% for 5%, and 2.3% to 12.5% for 6%. Even when this technique of dilution is used, the upper 95% limits are too high after three or four strokes or deaths, and the true limits and rates are even higher. It is clear that, if a surgeon reaches three or more events before the 100 CEAs have been performed, there needs to be some assessment of what might be wrong. The 100 CEAs minimum value may mask real problems with judgment, technique, or both.

As hospitals and institutions slowly but surely address the issue of individual surgeon outcomes and consider recertification for CEA privileges, the problem of low volume and inexperience will present a major hurdle in determining the adequacy of performance. The reason is the inability to obtain adequate statistical data on the basis of fewer than several hundred cases unless the outcomes are well above the minimum standards. One potential way to deal with this matter is to analyze the pooled results from a group of surgeons in a department or partnership. This compels senior surgeons to monitor and train their younger associates and partners.

PROSPECTIVE RANDOMIZED TRIALS COMPARING PRIMARY CLOSURE WITH PATCH ANGIOPLASTY RECONSTRUCTION

There are six published trials addressing this issue.[20-25] The authors of three studies conclude that there is no statistically significant difference in outcomes between the two types of closure, and the other three conclude that there is a difference. However, the *P* values for early postoperative internal carotid occlusion, 30-day stroke rates, and 50% or greater restenosis within the first postoperative year vary from 0.3 to 0.015. The real problem with interpreting the results of these six randomized prospective trials is the low power of the statistical tests that were used. *Power* quantifies the probability of detecting a real difference between two methods or treatments. It is the proportion of the test statistic (*P*) that falls below a certain chance of a type II error (false negative), usually $P < 0.05$, given that a method or treatment has a real effect. Put another way, the power of a test tells the likelihood that the hypothesis of no effect (or difference in outcome of two treatments) will be rejected when the treatment actually does have an effect (i.e., a true positive). For example, for a cutoff of 0.05 for statistical significance, power is the likelihood that, if the study were repeated with the same sample size in each cohort, the new *P* value still would be less than 0.05. The sample size plays a major role in determining power. In the most recent and statistically significant study,[25] for instance, the *P* values for a perioperative stroke ranged from 0.015 to 0.06 and, for early internal carotid occlusion, from 0.03 to 0.22. The powers computed from the data in the contingency tables ranged from 0.29 to 0.55, which yielded a cutoff value of 0.05. This means that, if the study were repeated with the same sample sizes, the chance of obtaining a $P < 0.05$ ranges from 29% to 55%, depending on the subset being tested. This illustration is typical (actually on the high side) of power values computed for strokes, occlusion, and early restenosis for the five other prospective randomized trials. The sample sizes simply are too small to detect 3% to 6% differences with adequate power.

An analysis of the pooled data from these six studies for the three end points of early postoperative occlusion, 30-day stroke rates, and 50% or greater restenosis in the first year is given in Table 3. The incidence of early internal carotid occlusion is 4.3% (20/462) for primary closure, 0.4% (1/242) for greater saphenous

TABLE 3.
Pooled Outcome Results for Six Prospective Randomized Studies Comparing Primary Closure With Patch Angioplasty Reconstruction

Outcomes	Primary Closure		Patch Angioplasty		*P*	Power ($\alpha = 0.05$)
	n	**% (95% CI)**	**n**	**% (95% CI)**		
Internal carotid occlusion in 30 days	20/462	4.3% (2.5% to 6.1%)	5/641	0.8% (0.2% to 1.4%)	0.001	0.90
Perioperative stroke in 30 days	18/462	3.9% (2.2% to 5.7%)	8/641	1.2% (0.2% to 2.0%)	0.008	0.83
≥50% restenosis in 1 year	33/448	7.4% (5.1% to 9.7%)	12/591	2.1% (0.9% to 3.1%)	<0.001	0.99

Note: Table adapted from References 20 through 25.
Abbreviation: CI, confidence interval.

vein patches, 1.0% (4/399) for other types of vein and synthetic patches, and 0.8% for all patched arteries. The *P* values are highly significant, but more importantly, the power (or probability of a true positive) is 0.99. That is, the chance of a type II statistical error is 1 – power = 0.01. Considering the many causes of a perioperative stroke, these results illustrate that the type of CEA reconstruction is a major, if not *the* major, independent variable. On the basis of these pooled data, patch reconstruction appears to have a threefold superiority to primary closure in terms of perioperative stroke prevention. Under these circumstances, it may be difficult in the future for adequately informed patients to agree to randomizing their operations between primary closure and patch reconstruction. The threefold difference between the 3.9% probability (95% CI, 2.1% to 5.7%) of a perioperative stroke with primary closure vs. 1.2% (95% CI, 0.3% to 2.1%) for patch reconstruction is enough to deter obligatory primary closure. Few patients would accept a flip of the coin that gives a 50-50 chance for a treatment associated with a risk of a perioperative stroke that is three times higher than the alternative treatment. Future prospective randomized trials of primary closure vs. patch reconstruction will be difficult to accomplish, and considering these data, they seem unnecessary. Like internal carotid occlusion and perioperative strokes, early 50% or greater restenosis (or, possibly, residual stenosis) is significantly and powerfully reduced by patching.

The results of these pooled data are compelling even though, taken individually, only three of the six studies concluded that patch reconstruction was superior to primary closure. Collectively, however, the probability of a false positive is very low, and the probability of a true positive is very high. Obligatory patching clearly is superior to obligatory primary closure.

OUTCOMES OF PROSPECTIVE RANDOMIZED AND NONRANDOMIZED STUDIES COMPARING PATCHING WITH PRIMARY CLOSURE

The pooled results of the 6 prospective randomized trials of patch angioplasty vs. primary closure that are presented in Table 3 can be expanded by considering nonrandomized studies containing a mix of primary closure and patch reconstruction. There are 3 nonrandomized studies that have data on early postoperative internal carotid occlusion,[26-28] 4 studies that have 30-day perioperative stroke data,[26-29] and 7 that contain data on 50% or greater restenosis in the first postoperative year.[26-32] Figure 1 illustrates the pooled results of the 9 studies (randomized and nonrandomized) with data on internal carotid occlusion; Figure 2 illustrates the pooled results of the 10 studies with perioperative stroke data; and

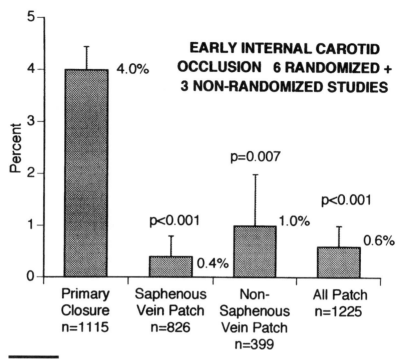

FIGURE 1.
The incidence of early postoperative internal carotid occlusion (thrombosis) for six randomized and three nonrandomized studies. The statistical power is greater than 0.99 for saphenous vein patch reconstruction vs. primary closure, 0.76 for nonsaphenous vein patches vs. primary closure, and greater than 0.99 for all patches vs. primary closure ($\alpha = 0.05$).

Figure 3 illustrates the pooled results of 13 studies with data regarding 50% or greater restenosis. These results are similar to those given in Table 3 for the 6 prospective randomized studies alone, with the exception that greater saphenous vein patches are associated with slightly better outcomes than alternative patches.

A recent analysis of long-term restenosis in 645 of the 720 patients undergoing CEAs in the ACAS strongly supports patch angioplasty over primary closure.[33] Depending on the cut point for the positive predictive value of the duplex scan data, the incidence of 60% or greater diameter restenosis was three- to fourfold lower for the 240 patched CEAs than for the 405 CEAs for which primary closure was performed ($P < 0.001$). Although randomization in the ACAS was between CEA and medical treatment, not the type of CEA reconstruction, this still is valuable information. Furthermore, there was no correlation of recurrent stenosis with other traditional risk factors, and the difference in restenosis

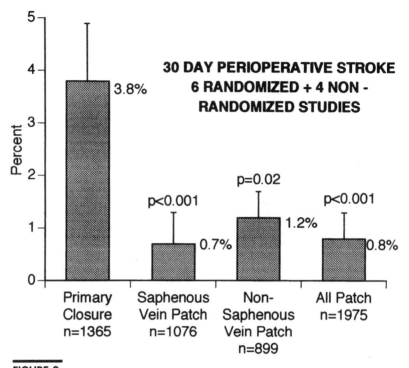

FIGURE 2.
The incidence of 30-day perioperative strokes for six randomized and four nonrandomized studies. The statistical power is 0.99 for greater saphenous vein patching vs. primary closure, 0.75 for nonsaphenous vein patches vs. primary closure, and greater than 0.99 for all patches vs. primary closure ($\alpha = 0.05$).

between primary closure and patch angioplasty remained highly significant even after correcting for covariants.

In my view, the data presented in Table 3 and in Figures 1 through 3 represent compelling evidence that obligatory primary closure simply does not give equivalent outcomes when compared with obligatory patch angioplasty. Although patch angioplasty does not necessarily need to be obligatory, it is strongly advisable to use it very frequently. For the past 15 years, I have reserved primary closure for arteriotomies that provide adequate exposure for obtaining a complete internal carotid artery end point limited to the bulb segment. This has occurred only in about 3% to 4% of my own series of CEAs. When, to obtain a complete end point, I have to extend the arteriotomy beyond the carotid bulb into the segment of the internal carotid artery that has a uniform diameter, I routinely use patch angioplasty, preferably with an autologous greater saphenous vein patch.

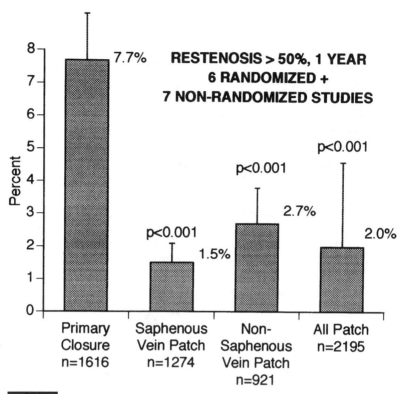

FIGURE 3.
The incidence of 50% or greater recurrent (or residual) stenosis in the first year after carotid endarterectomy for six randomized studies and seven nonrandomized studies. The power for saphenous veins, nonsaphenous veins, and all patch materials vs. primary closure is greater than 0.99 ($\alpha = 0.05$).

PRACTICAL AND THEORETICAL ADVANTAGES OF PATCH RECONSTRUCTION OVER PRIMARY CLOSURE

Surgeons who use patch angioplasty do so because it can make the reconstruction easier, it reduces the chance of a technical error, and most importantly, it provides reconstruction geometry that minimizes the risks for embolization, thrombosis, or recurrent stenosis. Patch angioplasty prevents the approximate 15% narrowing of the internal carotid artery distal to the bulb that is produced by primary closure. This adverse hemodynamic result is not always obvious to the operating surgeon. I recognized this problem 2 decades ago while removing the distal end of a Javid shunt after a long primary closure. Although the artery did not appear to have been narrowed, it was difficult to pull the shunt through the closure. Patch angioplasty can make reconstruction after a long or complex endarterectomy simple. It facilitates an aggressive approach to obtaining a complete feathered internal carotid end point by allowing a long arteriotomy without concern about stenosis produced by primary closure. Furthermore, patching expedites reconstruction after shortening of a redundant endarterectomized segment.[34] It allows the surgeon to optimize the carotid geometry; a gradual transition can be made from the common carotid bulb to the uniform diameter of the distal internal carotid artery.[35,36] Patching also facilitates repair of endarterectomy-produced common carotid "steps."[37] However, patch reconstruction does have some drawbacks that should be recognized. First, when it is used to close a tortuous or redundant endarterectomized segment, the tapered, patched segment straightens after flow has been restored and may produce a kink in the distal internal carotid artery or at the cephalad end of the patch itself. This can be prevented by internal carotid shortening.[34,35] My recent experience with shortening, however, has been that it increases the probability of early restenosis.[38] Second, patching increases carotid occlusion time by 5 to 6 minutes.[39]

The practical advantages of patching over primary closure have a theoretical basis. It is well accepted that residual atheromas and nonfeathered or nonsmooth endarterectomy transitions in the internal carotid artery (i.e., an incomplete end point) as well as large, concentric or eccentric common carotid steps can be harbingers of embolization, thrombosis, and restenosis.[40-44] These residual defects may produce markedly disturbed blood flow.[45] In addition, excessive "ballooning" of the carotid bulb, like the narrowing from primary closure, produces disturbed flow with low wall shear stresses and high wall shear stress gradients, both of which also are harbingers of restenosis.[46] Therefore, the final geometry of the patched segment should resemble the normal contour of the carotid artery as closely as possible.

Other potential disadvantages of patch reconstruction include the rare possibility of infection if synthetic patches are used and the serious problem of vein patch rupture. Central ruptures of greater saphenous vein patches have been reported to have an incidence of 0.5% to 4%.[47-51] Small diameter veins, ankle veins, and female sex have been implicated as contributing factors to patch rupture. However, it has recently been demonstrated that it is safe to use a greater saphenous vein having a distended diameter of 3.5 mm or more as a carotid patch.[52]

EFFECT OF PATCH MATERIAL ON OUTCOMES

The above meta-analysis of the six prospective randomized trials and nonrandomized studies of primary closure vs. patch reconstruction indicates that there is an absolute 3% to 4% potential for improvement in 30-day perioperative stroke rates by both obligatory and frequent patching. Moreover, when the perioperative stroke outcomes of studies containing a mix of primary closure and patching (selective patching) are superimposed on the stroke data for obligatory primary closure and obligatory patch reconstruction, there is an inverse linear relationship between the percentage of patch utilization and the incidence of perioperative strokes from nearly 4% for primary closure to only 1.2% for patching.[53] Considering that average combined perioperative stroke or death rates for CEA are in the range of 4% to 6%, the advantage of frequent or obligatory patch reconstruction is evident. A major unanswered question is which patch material or materials give the best protection against strokes and restenosis. There are a number of reports regarding the outcome for primary CEA that contain a mix of patch materials, including autologous greater saphenous veins, everted cervical veins, and two prostatic materials (polyethylene terephthalate [Dacron] and polytetrafluoroethylene [PTFE]). Although only one of these studies comes even close to a statistically significant difference in outcomes,[54] significant differences become apparent when the data are pooled.[55] Table 4 contains the 30-day perioperative stroke outcomes for autologous greater saphenous vein vs. synthetic patches (Dacron or PTFE),[21,25,29,34,39,54,56-58] saphenous vein vs. Dacron patches,[29,34,39,55,57] saphenous vein vs. PTFE patches,[21,25,29,58] and saphenous vein vs. everted cervical vein patches.[25,57,59] The large number of CEAs in the saphenous vein vs. synthetic patch data gives a narrow 95% CI and indicates that saphenous vein patching is associated with an excellent perioperative stroke rate of 1.2%, which is about half the rate of 2.7% for synthetic patching. The probability of a false-negative observation is remote ($P < 0.001$), and the likelihood of a true-positive association is very high (power = 0.98). Similarly, saphenous vein patches clearly are superior to Dacron patches in terms of perioperative strokes. The mean values of perioperative stroke rates for saphenous vein and PTFE patches are comparable, but the P and power values are not statistically significant because of smaller case numbers. The comparison between saphenous vein patches and everted cervical vein patches is weaker. Nevertheless, two of these three studies were published by the same group of surgeons,[57,59] and the stroke rate for saphenous vein patches is higher (1.7%) than is the case in the third study (1.2%). An autologous greater saphenous vein appears to be the patch material of choice in comparison with synthetics, and probably also in comparison with an everted cervical vein, although the latter may be shown in the future to be an acceptable alternative material for autologous patching.

A similar analysis of the 50% or greater restenosis rate at 1 year is given in Table 5. Greater saphenous vein patches clearly are

TABLE 4.
Pooled Data Analysis for 30-Day Perioperative Stroke Rate for Greater Saphenous Vein Patching vs. Synthetic Patching and Everted Cervical Vein Patching During CEA

References	n	% (95% CI)	n	% (95% CI)	P	Power
		Saphenous Vein Patch		Synthetic Patch (Dacron Plus PTFE)		
(1) 21,25,29,34, 39,54,56-58	28/2,242	1.2% (0.7 to 1.7%)	73/2,733	2.7% (2.7% to 6.0%)	<0.001	0.98
		Saphenous Vein Patch		Dacron Patch		
(2) 29,34,39,56,57	16/1,332	1.2% (0.6% to 1.8%)	30/1,015	3.0% (2.0% to 4.0%)	0.004	0.81
		Saphenous Vein Patch		PTFE Patch		
(3) 21,25,29,58	5/650	0.8% (0.1% to 1.5%)	11/541	2.0% (0.8% to 3.2%)	0.096	0.38
		Saphenous Vein Patch		Everted Cervical Vein Patch		
(4) 25,57,59	6/354	1.7% (0.4% to 3.0%)	5/252	2.0% (0.3% to 3.7%)	0.96	N/A

Abbreviations: CEA, carotid endarterectomy; *CI*, confidence interval; *PTFE*, polytetrafluoroethylene; *N/A*, not applicable.

TABLE 5.
Pooled Data Analysis for 50% or Greater Restenosis at 1 Year for Greater Saphenous Vein Patching vs. Synthetic Patching and Everted Cervical Vein Patching During CEA

References	n	% (95% CI)	n	% (95% CI)	P	Power
(1)21,25,29,34, 39,57,58	Saphenous Vein Patch		Synthetic Patch (Dacron + PTFE)			
	15/1,246	1.2% (0.6% to 1.8%)	50/1,228	4.1% (3.0% to 5.2%)	<0.001	0.99
(2)29,34,39,57	Saphenous Vein Patch		Dacron Patch			
	12/915	1.3% (0.6% to 2.0%)	40/732	5.5% (3.9% to 7.1%)	0.001	0.99
(3)25,29,57	Saphenous Vein Patch		PTFE Patch			
	5/563	0.9% (0.2% to 1.7%)	10/474	2.1% (0.8% to 3.4%)	0.17	0.28
(4)25,57,59	Saphenous Vein Patch		Everted Cervical Vein Patch			
	12/346	3.5% (1.6% to 5.4%)	13/241	5.4% (2.6% to 8.2%)	0.36	N/A

Note: $P = 0.008$, Power = 0.85 for saphenous vein patching in nine studies with synthetic patches vs. the three studies using everted cervical veins.
Abbreviations: CEA, carotid endarterectomy; *CI*, confidence interval; *PTFE*, polytetrafluoroethylene; *N/A*, not applicable.

superior to synthetic patches in general and to Dacron patches in particular. Although the recurrence rate when using PTFE patches is twice that for when using saphenous vein patches, the 95% CIs are wide and the difference is not statistically significant. However, as with perioperative strokes, the chance of a type II statistical error is high. Interestingly, as with the stroke data, the restenosis rate for a saphenous vein patch is higher than expected in the studies in which it is compared with an everted cervical vein patch ($P = 0.008$). An autologous saphenous vein again appears to be the optimal patch material to use to avoid recurrent carotid stenosis.

I recently have completed an analysis of the outcomes for 370 CEAs performed with saphenous vein patches compared with another 308 CEAs with Dacron patches.[38] Cox proportional hazards analysis indicated significantly higher risk ratios for restenosis when using Dacron than when using vein patches (3.0 with a 95% CI of 1.6 to 6.8). On the basis of this personal experience and the pooled analysis of greater saphenous vein vs. Dacron patch angioplasty presented in Table 5, I have abandoned routine use of Dacron as a patch material unless an autologous vein is not available. The minimal extra time, effort, and minor morbidity associated with autologous greater saphenous vein harvesting are well worth it.

CONCLUSION

The stroke and combined stroke and death outcomes of CEA for randomized trials and regional, statewide, and pooled studies approach or overlap the recommended maximum 6% threshold for symptomatic carotid lesions and the 3% threshold for asymptomatic carotid stenosis. Recent regional and statewide studies suggest that perioperative outcomes are improving. However, they are a long way from the best possible 0.5% perioperative stroke rate and 1% combined perioperative stroke and death rates. The variance among individual surgeon's results is concerning, as is the inability to clearly define the operative risk for the patients of low-volume or inexperienced surgeons. Highly frequent or obligatory patch angioplasty, especially when done with an autologous greater saphenous vein, offers an opportunity to obtain acceptable or even gold standard results. Surgeons with an undefined track record or one that is known to be marginal or even poor should strongly consider patching. The 30-day perioperative stroke rate of 0.7% to 1.2% and the 1-year 50% or greater restenosis rate of 1.2% to 2.1% for patch angioplasty with autologous greater saphenous vein patches in the studies presented herein should serve as a benchmark for other types of CEA reconstruction and/or the use of other patch materials, as well as for catheter-based carotid balloon angioplasty with or without stenting.

REFERENCES

1. North American Symptomatic Carotid Endarterectomy Trial Collaborators: Beneficial effect of carotid endarterectomy in symptomatic patients with high-grade carotid stenosis. *N Engl J Med* 325:445-453, 1991.
2. Barnett HJM, Taylor DW, Eliasziw M, et al: Benefit of carotid endarterectomy in patients with symptomatic moderate or severe stenosis. *N Engl J Med* 339:1415-1425, 1998.
3. Executive Committee for the Asymptomatic Carotid Atherosclerosis Study: Endarterectomy for asymptomatic carotid artery stenosis. *JAMA* 273:1421-1428, 1995.
4. Ad Hoc Committee, Society for Vascular Surgery and NA- ISCVS: Carotid endarterectomy: Practice guidelines. *J Vasc Surg* 15:469-479, 1992.
5. Ad Hoc Committee, American Heart Association: Guidelines for carotid endarterectomy. *Stroke* 26:188-201, 1995.
6. Young B, Moore WS, Robertson JT, et al: An analysis of perioperative surgical mortality and morbidity in the Asymptomatic Carotid Atherosclerosis Study. *Stroke* 27:2216-2224, 1996.
7. Biller J, Feinberg WM, Castaldo JE, et al: Guidelines for carotid endarterectomy. Stroke Council, American Heart Association. *Stroke* 29:554-562, 1998.
8. Hertzer NR: A personal view: The Asymptomatic Carotid Atherosclerosis Study results—read the label carefully. *J Vasc Surg* 23:167-171, 1996.
9. Riles TS, Imparato AM, Jacobowitz GR, et al: The cause of perioperative stroke after carotid endarterectomy. *J Vasc Surg* 19:206-216, 1994.
10. Archie JP: Management of acute postendarterectomy neurological deficits, in Whittemore AD (ed): *Advances in Vascular Surgery,* vol 3. Chicago, Mosby, 1995, pp 97-114.
11. Kucey DS, Bowyer B, Iron K, et al: Determinants of outcome after carotid endarterectomy. *J Vasc Surg* 28:1051-1058, 1998.
12. Mayo SW, Eldrup-Jorgensen J, Lucas FL, et al: Carotid endarterectomy after NASCET and ACAS: A statewide study. *J Vasc Surg* 27:1017-1023, 1998.
13. Perler BA, Dardik A, Burleyson GP, et al: Influence of age and hospital volume on the results of carotid endarterectomy: A statewide analysis of 9918 cases. *J Vasc Surg* 27:25-33, 1998.
14. Yates GW, Bergamini TM, George SM, et al: Carotid endarterectomy results from a state vascular society. *Am J Surg* 173:342-344, 1997.
15. Ruby ST, Robinson D, Lynch JT, et al: Outcome analysis of carotid endarterectomy in Connecticut: The impact of volume and specialty. *Ann Vasc Surg* 10:22-26, 1996.
16. Goldstein LB, Samsa GP, Matchar DB, et al: Multicenter review of perioperative risk factors for endarterectomy for asymptomatic carotid artery stenosis. *Stroke* 29:750-753, 1998.

17. Rothwell PM, Slattery J, Warlow CP: A systematic review of the risks of stroke and death due to endarterectomy for symptomatic carotid stenosis. *Stroke* 27:260-265, 1996.
18. Rothwell PM, Slattery J, Warlow CP: A systematic comparison of the risks of stroke and death due to carotid endarterectomy for symptomatic and asymptomatic patients. *Stroke* 27:266-269, 1996.
19. Hanna EL, Popp AJ, Tranmer B, et al: Relationship between provider volume and mortality for carotid endarterectomy in New York State. *Stroke* 29:2292-2297, 1998.
20. Eikelboom BC, Ackerstaff RGA, Hoeneveld H, et al: Benefits of carotid patching: A randomized study. *J Vasc Surg* 7:240-247, 1998.
21. Lord RSA, Raj TB, Stary DL, et al: Comparison of saphenous vein patch, polytetrafluoroethylene patch, and direct arteriotomy closure after carotid endarterectomy: Part I. Perioperative results. *J Vasc Surg* 9:521-529, 1989.
22. Clagett GP, Patterson CB, Fisher DF, et al: Vein patch versus primary closure for carotid endarterectomy: A randomized prospective study in a selected group of patients. *J Vasc Surg* 9:213-223, 1989.
23. Katz D, Snyder SO, Gandhi RH, et al: Long-term follow-up for recurrent stenosis: A prospective randomized study of expanded polytetrafluoroethylene patch angioplasty versus primary closure after carotid endarterectomy. *J Vasc Surg* 19:198-205, 1994.
24. Vascular Research Group: Randomized controlled trial of patch angioplasty for carotid endarterectomy. *Br J Surg* 80:1528-1530, 1993.
25. AbuRahma AF, Khan JH, Robinson PA, et al: Prospective randomized trial of carotid endarterectomy with primary closure and patch angioplasty with saphenous vein, jugular vein, and polytetrafluoroethylene: Perioperative (30-day) results. *J Vasc Surg* 24:998-1008, 1996.
26. Little JR, Bryerton BS, Furlan AJ: Saphenous vein patch grafts in carotid endarterectomy. *J Neurosurg* 61:743-747, 1984.
27. Archie J: Prevention of early restenosis and thrombosis occlusion after carotid endarterectomy by saphenous vein patch angioplasty. *Stroke* 17:901-905, 1986.
28. Hertzer NR, Beven EG, O'Hara PJ, et al: A prospective study of vein patch angioplasty during carotid endarterectomy. *Ann Surg* 206:628-635, 1987.
29. Rosenthal D, Archie JP, Garcia-Rinaldi R, et al: Carotid patch angioplasty: Immediate and long-term results. *J Vasc Surg* 12:326-333, 1990.
30. Katz MM, Jones GT, Degenhardt J: The use of patch angioplasty to alter the incidence of carotid restenosis following thromboendarterectomy. *J Cardiovasc Surg* 28:2-8, 1987.
31. Ouriel K, Green R: Clinical and technical factors influencing recurrent carotid stenosis and occlusion after endarterectomy. *J Vasc Surg* 5:702-706, 1987.
32. Ten Holder JBM, Ackerstaff RGA, Thoe Schwartzenberg GWS, et al: The impact of vein patch angioplasty on long-term surgical outcome of carotid endarterectomy. *J Cardiovasc Surg* 31:58-65, 1990.
33. Moore WS, Kempczinski RF, Nelson JJ, et al: Recurrent carotid steno-

sis: Results of the Asymptomatic Carotid Atherosclerosis Study. *Stroke* 29:2018-2025, 1998.

34. Goldman KA, Su WT, Riles TS, et al: A comparative study of saphenous vein, internal jugular vein, and knitted Dacron patches for carotid endarterectomy. *Ann Vasc Surg* 9:71-79, 1985.

35. Archie JP: Carotid endarterectomy with reconstruction techniques tailored to operative findings. *J Vasc Surg* 17:141-151, 1993.

36. Archie JP: Geometric dimension changes with carotid endarterectomy reconstruction. *J Vasc Surg* 25:488-498, 1997.

37. Archie JP: The endarterectomy produced common carotid artery step: A harbinger of early emboli and late restenosis. *J Vasc Surg* 23:932-939, 1996.

38. Archie JP: Carotid endarterectomy outcome with vein or Dacron patch angioplasty and internal carotid shortening. *J Vasc Surg*, 29:654-664, 1999.

39. Archie JP: The occlusion and shunt times for carotid endarterectomy with primary closure, patch angioplasty and adjunctive reconstructive procedures. *J Vasc Surg* 33:141-150, 1999.

40. Sawchuk AP, Flanigan DP, Machi J, et al: The fate of unrepaired minor technical defects detected by intraoperative ultrasonography during carotid endarterectomy. *J Vasc Surg* 9:671-676, 1989.

41. Green RM, McNamera JA, Ouriel K, et al: The clinical course of residual carotid arterial disease. *J Vasc Surg* 13:112-120, 1991.

42. O'Donnell TF Jr, Callow AD, Scott G, et al: Ultrasound characteristics of recurrent carotid disease: Hypothesis explaining the low incidence of symptomatic recurrence. *J Vasc Surg* 2:26-41, 1985.

43. Clagett GP, Robinowitz M, Youkey JR, et al: Morphogenesis and clinicopathologic characteristics of recurrent carotid disease. *J Vasc Surg* 3:10-23, 1986.

44. Reilly LM, Okuhn SP, Rapp JH, et al: Recurrent carotid stenosis: A consequence of local or systemic factors: The influence of unrepaired technical defects. *J Vasc Surg* 11:448-460, 1990.

45. Bandyk DR, Kaebnick NW, Adams MD, et al: Turbulence occurring after carotid bifurcation endarterectomy: A harbinger of residual and recurrent carotid stenosis. *J Vasc Surg* 7:261-274, 1988.

46. Wells DR, Archie JP, Kleinstreuer C: The effect of carotid artery geometry on the magnitude and distribution of wall shear stress gradient. *J Vasc Surg* 23:667-678, 1996.

47. Riles TS, Lamparello PJ, Giangola G, et al: Rupture of the vein patch: A rare complication of carotid endarterectomy. *Surgery* 107:10-12, 1990.

48. Archie JP, Green JJ: Saphenous vein rupture pressure, rupture stress, and carotid endarterectomy vein patch reconstruction. *Surgery* 107:389-396, 1990.

49. Tawes RL, Treiman RL: Vein patch rupture after carotid endarterectomy: A survey of the Western Vascular Society members. *Ann Vasc Surg* 5:71-73, 1991.

50. O'Hara PJ, Hertzer NR, Krajewski LP, et al: Saphenous vein patch rupture after carotid endarterectomy. *J Vasc Surg* 15:504-509, 1992.

51. Scott EW, Dolson L, Day AL, et al: Carotid endarterectomy complicated by vein patch rupture. *Neurosurgery* 31:373-377, 1992.
52. Archie JP: Carotid endarterectomy saphenous vein patch rupture revisited: Selective utilization based on vein diameter. *J Vasc Surg* 24:346-351, 1996.
53. Archie JP: Patching with carotid endarterectomy: When to do it and what to use, in Rutherford RB (ed): *Seminars in Vascular Surgery*, vol II. Philadelphia, W.B. Saunders, Company, 1998, pp 24-29.
54. Hertzer NR, O'Hara PJ, Mascha EJ, et al: Early outcome assessment for 2228 consecutive carotid endarterectomy procedures: The Cleveland Clinic experience from 1989 to 1995. *J Vasc Surg* 25:1-10, 1997.
55. Archie JP: Carotid patching: What is the optimal patch material? in Goldstone J (ed): *Perspective in Vascular Surgery*, vol 10, New York, Thieme Medical Publishers, Inc., 1999, pp 105-112.
56. Fode NC, Sundt TM, Robertson JT, et al: Multicenter retrospective review of results and complications of carotid endarterectomy in 1981. *Stroke* 17:370-376, 1986.
57. Jacobowitz GR, Kalish JA, Lee AM, et al: Long-term follow-up of saphenous vein, internal jugular vein and knitted Dacron patches for carotid endarterectomy. *Stroke* 29:333-337, 1998.
58. Allen PH, Jackson MR, O'Donnell SD, et al: Saphenous vein versus polytetrafluoroethylene carotid patch angioplasty. *Am J Surg* 174:115-117, 1997.
59. Dardik H, Wolodiger F, Silverstri F, et al: Clinical experience with everted cervical vein as patch material after carotid endarterectomy. *J Vasc Surg* 25:545-553, 1997.

CHAPTER 2

Decision Making for Asymptomatic Patients With Critical Carotid Stenosis

James M. Estes, M.D.
Assistant Professor of Surgery, Tufts University School of Medicine, Staff Surgeon, New England Medical Center, Boston, Massachusetts

Carotid endarterectomy (CEA) was first introduced in 1954 as a treatment for an ischemic stroke. Enthusiasm for this operation grew until 1985, when over 100,000 CEAs were performed in the United States. Thereafter, prompted by concerns of improper patient selection, questionable results, and complications, a decrease in CEA rates of more than 30% occurred by 1990.[1] Despite the availability of positive data from randomized prospective studies,[2,3] doubts still remain regarding the efficacy of CEA for the asymptomatic patient. Because these studies demonstrate a margin of benefit from CEA for asymptomatic patients that is much less than for symptomatic patients, it is presumed that other factors that may affect outcome take on greater significance when considering CEA for asymptomatic patients. These include patient demographics, co-morbidity, the experience and the results of individual surgeons, and the hospital setting in which the operation is performed.

IMPACT OF PROSPECTIVE RANDOMIZED TRIALS

The efficacy of CEA for asymptomatic patients with carotid bifurcation atherosclerosis has been addressed in the Veterans Affairs Cooperative Study[3] (VACS) and the Asymptomatic Carotid Atherosclerosis Study[2] (ACAS). VACS randomized 444 men with asymptomatic carotid lesions with greater than 50% stenosis to surgery or medical management. They found that neurologic events (i.e., strokes and transient ischemic attacks) in the surgical group were reduced from 21% to 8%. However, the study was widely criticized not only because of its failure to demonstrate a long-term reduction in the occurrence of ipsilateral strokes but also because of its small sample size. ACAS examined 1,662 randomized patients and demonstrated stroke/mortality rates of 5% in the operated group vs. 11% for medically treated patients during a 5-year period. The perioperative stroke and death rates were 2.4% and 1.9%, respectively, and, in the analysis of the trial, the authors acknowledged that low perioperative morbidity and mortality rates are required to confer the small benefit from surgery in these patients. In addition, the external validity of the ACAS data have been criticized because only centers documenting excellent results were invited to enroll patients: a survey of 1,511 CEAs performed outside the study by ACAS participating surgeons documented stroke/mortality rates of 1.7%.[4]

Demographic data from VACS and ACAS underscore the prevalence of serious medical co-morbidity in this population. In particular, coronary artery disease was the most common medical risk factor, identified in 58% and 69% of patients in VACS and ACAS, respectively. The impact of cardiovascular disease in both studies was reflected in the mortality statistics: 20% of deaths in VACS and 49% in ACAS were due to cardiac causes, and myocardial infarction accounted for about half. Therefore, in asymptomatic patients, the prevalence of pre-existing coronary artery disease and its contribution to postoperative death by myocardial infarction may be among the major factors that determine the outcome and benefits of CEA.

IMPACT OF DEMOGRAPHICS AND CO-MORBIDITY

The benefits of CEA in asymptomatic patients are realized over time. Those patients with significant co-morbidity and increased operative risk or diminished life expectancy may not have a significant reduction in their risk of a stroke or death. These issues are addressed in a multidisciplinary consensus statement from the American Heart Association.[5] The authors state that CEA for asymptomatic patients with critical carotid stenosis is appropriate if the stroke/mortality rates are less than 3% and inappropriate if the stroke/mortality rates are more than 6%.

In addition to coronary artery disease, carotid atherosclerosis in patients has been associated with a high prevalence of other illnesses such as hypertension and diabetes mellitus (DM)[6] and attempts have been made to quantify the impact of these co-morbidities and other factors on outcome after CEA. A recent study found that death within 3 years after CEA was associated with ischemic heart disease and DM.[7] In another report, Akbari and colleagues[8] studied 732 patients with a 39% prevalence of DM and found no differences in perioperative outcomes. They did note an increased prevalence of cardiac disease among patients with diabetes as well as a greater incidence of nonfatal cardiac complications but did not report long-term follow-up data in this population. Perler[9] examined the outcomes after CEA in elderly patients and found no difference in early results with respect to age, but long-term data were not available. Eagle et al.[10] analyzed the incidence of perioperative cardiac complications in patients undergoing vascular surgery and identified advanced age, DM, active angina pectoris, and ventricular ectopy as independent risk factors for adverse cardiac events.

Many of the aforementioned recent studies document admirably low complication rates after CEA. Because a stroke or death after CEA is an infrequent event, most studies have insufficient numbers of patients with those endpoints to adequately examine the association between co-morbidity and adverse events.

To overcome this problem, we examined the impact of co-morbidity and demographic factors on early and late outcomes after CEA using a large sample of Medicare beneficiaries. We focused on the presence of common risk factors associated with atherosclerosis along with age, demographic variables, other co-morbid conditions, and hospital characteristics to assess their impact on early strokes and death (i.e., within 30 days of CEA) and on late mortality. Using multivariate logistic regression and proportional hazards regression models, we quantified the relative contributions of each parameter for the endpoints examined.[11]

We selected our sample from the Health Care Financing Administration (HCFA) Medical Provider Analysis and Review files, which contain a random sample of approximately 20% of all Medicare beneficiaries with Part A coverage during 1988, 1989, and 1990. Each record in the data set represents an admission to a hospital and contains up to five diagnostic codes and up to three procedure codes. We also obtained each patient's age, race, sex, and state of residence from this data set.

We sampled patients 66 years of age or older with an International Classification of Diseases-ninth revision-Clinical Modification (ICD-9-CM) procedure code of 38.12 (i.e., endarterectomy of vessels of the head and neck other than intracranial vessels) and a diagnosis code of 433 (i.e., occlusion or stenosis of the precerebral arteries) in the calendar years 1988, 1989, and 1990 (N = 23,730). After exclusions, 22,165 patients met eligibility criteria (Table 1).

TABLE 1.

Patients Excluded From Analysis

Reason	Number	Percent of Original Sample
Race unknown or other	937	3.9
No coding for carotid stenosis	598	2.5
CEA during previous year (1988 patients)	162	0.7
No information on hospital teaching status	47	0.2
Date of death unknown	14	<0.1
No information on number of hospital beds	11	<0.1
Missing other data	15	<0.1
Total	**1,625***	**6.8**

*Some patients were missing more than one parameter.
Abbreviation: CEA, carotid endarterectomy.

CHARACTERISTICS OF PATIENT SAMPLE

Table 2 outlines the demographic and co-morbid characteristics of the study population. There was a slight preponderance of men (56.7%). Nearly 10% were seen with recent strokes, and 16.6% had transient ischemic attack (TIA) as one of the admitting diagnoses, representing a combined proportion of 26.2% for patients with symptomatic carotid disease. Hypertension (34.8%), DM (14.6%), cardiovascular disease (28%), and congestive heart failure (CHF) (3.7%) were the major co-morbid conditions coded in the admitting diagnoses. Patients who underwent simultaneous coronary bypass and CEA procedures (2.1%) represented a small sample of the group. The geographic region with the largest number of patients was the Southeast (38.4%), and the smallest was the Northeast (15.8%).

We used logistic regression analysis to examine the influence of acute myocardial infarction (AMI), CHF, and coronary artery bypass graft surgery during the index admission on both death and the occurrence of a stroke within 30 days of the index procedure. Other covariates in the models included patient demographic characteristics, indication for surgery, other co-morbid conditions, and hospital characteristics. The reported odds ratios were adjusted for all variables in the models.

PERIOPERATIVE MORBIDITY AND MORTALITY

Overall, the rates of strokes and death within 30 days of operation were 2.4% and 2.3%, respectively, representing a combined rate of 4.7%. Table 3 shows the relationship between demographic and

TABLE 2.
Prevalence of Demographic and Co-morbidity Variables in
Medicare Patients Undergoing Carotid Endarterectomy

Variable	Number	Percent
Age 66–70 years	6,959	31.4
Age 71–75 years	7,365	33.2
Age 76–80 years	5,153	23.2
Age older than 80 years	2,688	12.1
Female sex	9,587	43.3
Black race	538	2.4
Hypertension	7,711	34.8
Diabetes mellitus	3,242	14.6
Atherosclerosis	1,357	6.1
Acute myocardial infarction	315	1.4
CHF	817	3.7
Other cardiovascular disease	5,993	27.0
Malignancy	448	2.0
TIA or amaurosis	3,680	16.6
Recent stroke	2,122	9.6
CAB with CEA	457	2.1
Geographic region:		
West	3,242	14.6
Northeast	3,508	15.8
Southeast	8,501	38.4
Midwest	6,279	28.3

Abbreviations: CHF, congestive heart failure; *TIA*, transient ischemic attack; *CEA*, carotid endarterectomy; *CAB*, coronary artery bypass.

co-morbidity parameters and the likelihood of a perioperative stroke. Controlling for all other variables, we found that patients seen with acute strokes had more than a fivefold increased likelihood of early postoperative strokes. Patients with DM, AMI, and CHF were 32%, 71%, and 80% more likely, respectively, to have early strokes than other patients without these diagnoses. Although there was a trend toward increased stroke risk with age, this reached statistical significance only with the group aged 76 to 80 years. These patients were 30% more likely than others to experience postoperative strokes. There was no difference in perioperative stroke rates based on hospital teaching status or geographic region (data not shown).

Advanced age and co-morbidity had a greater impact on the likelihood of perioperative death (Table 4). For patients older than 75 years, the odds of death increased by 50% and were doubled for

TABLE 3.
Impact of Age, Sex, Race, and Co-morbidity on Perioperative Strokes After Carotid Endarterectomy

Parameter	Adjusted Odds Ratio	95% Confidence Interval
Age 71-75 years	1.079	0.859-1.355
Age 76-80 years	1.298*	1.024-1.646
Age 81 years and older	1.130	0.839-1.523
Race: black vs. white	1.165	0.694-1.955
Female vs. male	1.165	0.975-1.393
Diabetes	1.329*	1.054-1.677
CHF	1.699†	1.171-2.466
Hypertension	1.008	0.833-1.220
Acute myocardial infarction	1.714	0.970-3.028
Other cardiovascular disease	0.896	0.721-1.112
Malignancy	1.351	0.781-2.339
Recent stroke	5.439‡	4.461-6.631
CEA with CAB	0.943	0.470-1.890

Note: Odds ratios are adjusted for covariates. Age categories are compared with patients 65 to 70 years old.
*Indicates statistical significance (chi-squared $P < 0.05$).
†$P < 0.01$.
‡$P < 0.001$.
Abbreviations: CHF, congestive heart failure; CEA, carotid endarterectomy; CAB, coronary artery bypass.

those older than 80 years. Patients seen with acute strokes had a 3.5-fold greater likelihood of perioperative death. Active cardiac disease conferred the greatest risk of perioperative mortality: patients with AMI were nine times more likely to die and those with CHF were three times more likely to die in the postoperative period than those patients without these diagnoses. Patients with DM had a 29% increased likelihood of death, whereas a diagnosis of hypertension was associated with a reduced incidence of perioperative mortality after CEA. Combined CEA and coronary artery bypass procedures increased the perioperative death rate threefold. There was no difference in perioperative death rates based on hospital teaching status or geographic region (data not shown).

LONG-TERM FOLLOW-UP

The sample of Medicare beneficiaries undergoing CEA during the years 1988 through 1990 was followed for a mean period of 3.1

TABLE 4.

Impact of Age, Sex, Race, and Co-morbidity on Perioperative Death After Carotid Endarterectomy

Parameter	Adjusted Odds Ratio	95% Confidence Interval
Age 71-75 years	1.182	0.924-1.511
Age 76-80 years	1.499[*]	1.163-1.933
Age 81 years and older	2.174[†]	1.643-2.876
Race: black vs. white	1.429	0.827-2.469
Female vs. male	0.898	0.745-1.083
Diabetes	1.330[‡]	1.044-1.696
CHF	3.085[†]	2.334-4.077
Hypertension	0.641[†]	0.513-0.801
Acute myocardial infarction	9.050[†]	6.631-12.351
Other cardiovascular disease	0.946	0.761-1.176
Malignancy	2.235[†]	1.431-3.491
Recent stroke	3.589[†]	2.911-4.425
CEA with CAB	3.260[†]	2.214-4.799

Note: Odds ratios for age categories are compared with patients 65 to 70 years old.
[*]$P < 0.01$.
[†]$P < 0.001$.
[‡]Indicates statistical significance (chi-squared $P < 0.05$).
Abbreviations: CHF, congestive heart failure; *CEA*, carotid endarterectomy; *CAB*, coronary artery bypass.

years. During this sampling interval, 6,132 patients died, representing 27.7% of the total.

The results of the proportional hazards model are shown in Table 5. The effects of age were roughly linear with respect to death rates during the follow-up period, such that those patients older than 80 years had more than a twofold greater chance of dying. Women were 25% less likely to die than men.

Cardiac co-morbidity had a substantial impact on late outcomes. CHF represented the most significant risk factor for late death; the hazard ratio was 2.73. AMI conferred a similar risk of long-term death (hazard ratio, 2.40), and DM conferred a 51% increase in the risk of late death. As observed with the results of perioperative mortality, a diagnosis of hypertension appeared to confer improved long-term survival after CEA. Malignancies were present in 2% of the sample and were associated with a twofold increase in the long-term death rate. The performance of simulta-

TABLE 5.
Impact of Age, Sex, Race, and Co-morbidity on Late Death After
Carotid Endarterectomy

Parameter	Hazard Ratio	95% Confidence Interval
Age 71-75 years	1.250[*]	1.168-1.337
Age 76-80 years	1.537[*]	1.432-1.649
Age 81 years and older	2.161[*]	1.996-2.339
Race: black vs. white	1.187[†]	1.017-1.385
Female vs. male	0.752[*]	0.713-0.792
Diabetes	1.519[*]	1.423-1.621
CHF	2.569[*]	2.331-2.831
Hypertension	0.865[*]	0.818-0.915
Acute myocardial infarction	2.405[*]	2.066-2.801
Other cardiovascular disease	1.025	0.967-1.086
Malignancy	2.112[*]	1.844-2.420
Recent stroke	1.513[*]	1.402-1.632
CEA with CAB	1.060	0.891-1.261

Note: Hazard ratios for age categories are compared with patients 65 to 70 years old.
[*]$P < 0.001$.
[†]Indicates statistical significance (chi-squared $P < 0.05$).
Abbreviations: CHF, congestive heart failure; CEA, carotid endarterectomy; CAB,
coronary artery bypass.

neous CEA and a coronary artery bypass, which was associated
with greater perioperative mortality, had no impact on long-term
survival. There was no difference in late outcomes based on hospital teaching status or geographic region (data not shown).

CONCLUSIONS

CAROTID ENDARTERECTOMY OUTCOME AND CARDIAC DISEASE

We found that active cardiovascular disease was a prominent risk
factor for poor perioperative and long-term outcomes. AMI
increased the likelihood of perioperative and late death by factors
of 9.0 and 2.4, respectively, and CHF contributed to an increased
likelihood of early and late death by factors of 3.1 and 2.6, respectively. The small group of patients who underwent a combined
coronary artery bypass and CEA had increased perioperative mortality (likely due to the coronary artery bypass) but no increase in
late death rates.

It is unclear why CHF contributes to an increased stroke rate
after CEA. It may be a marker for more severe and diffuse cerebrovascular disease, or it may be a sign that indicates those

patients with atrial arrhythmias who are at increased risk for an embolic stroke. Plecha and associates[12] documented similar findings in a series of nearly 10,000 CEAs.

CAROTID ENDARTERECTOMY OUTCOME AND OTHER CO-MORBIDITIES

DM was associated with a 33% increase in the perioperative death rate, and malignancies were associated with more than a twofold increase in the risk of perioperative death after CEA (Table 4). A recent stroke also increased the risk of perioperative death by a factor of 3.5. These variables also contributed to significantly reduced long-term survival rates (Table 5).

Interestingly, hypertension was associated with a reduced risk of early and late mortality after CEA. There are several explanations for this paradoxical observation. First, the Medicare database from 1988 through 1990 captured only five diagnostic codes, including the primary diagnosis mandating hospital admission. Therefore, the potential for coding bias and omission exists when the patient's medical record is examined. Jencks et al.[13] from the HCFA have documented undercoding of chronic illnesses in hospitalized patients, especially hypertension, which was associated with inexplicably lower than average in-hospital death rates. They concluded that chronic illnesses with a high prevalence, such as hypertension, are subject to coding omissions and bias when insurance claims forms are prepared. Presumably, patients with fewer co-morbidities are more likely to have hypertension coded, thus accounting for the improved outcome. Undercoding was presumed in our study because the incidence of hypertension (34%) was significantly less than the 50% to 60% incidence documented in the North American Symptomatic Carotid Endarterectomy Trial (NASCET),[6] in ACAS,[2] and in another large series.[14]

We observed that CHF had a strong negative impact on perioperative outcome and late survival. This diagnostic code was present in 3.7% of our study group, which is similar to the 5% incidence documented in VACS.[3] Also, 15% of our sample had the diagnostic code for DM compared with 19% in NASCET. We therefore concluded that diagnostic coding for DM and CHF was more consistently applied compared with hypertension in our patient sample.

CAROTID ENDARTERECTOMY OUTCOME AND AGE

Increasing age was also associated with increased perioperative death rates after CEA. This finding was significant for patients older than 76 years and especially for those older than 80 years, who had a twofold increased rate of death after surgery (Table 4).

Long-term data also demonstrated similarly increased risks of death among the older population (Table 5).

COMMENTS

In our study, 26% of patients undergoing CEA had a diagnostic code for a recent stroke, transient cerebral ischemia, or amaurosis fugax (Table 2). Other contemporaneous reports highlight the lower than expected proportion of symptomatic patients observed in our study. For example, in 1989, Callow and Mackey[14] reported the results of CEA in 619 patients, 71% of whom were symptomatic. We considered coding omissions during preparation of the claims forms as one potential cause for these results. Undercoding of chronic illnesses, such as hypertension, has been documented in Medicare patients[13] and is discussed above. However, of the five diagnostic codes available in our patient database, the first code is reserved for the primary diagnosis prompting hospital admission. Because hospital compensation is related to the diagnosis-related group (DRG) classification, it seems less likely that a TIA or stroke code would be omitted from the admitting diagnostic process than a code for a chronic illness such as hypertension.

We assume that our data are subject to some undercoding bias related to the symptoms seen on admission. However, the consistency of the CEA rates for asymptomatic disease across geographic regions (data not shown) and hospital types suggests that many more CEAs were performed for asymptomatic disease between 1988 and 1990 than were previously reported.

Our results regarding the impact of a recent stroke on outcome also warrant further discussion. The stroke rate for patients with an admitting diagnostic code for a recent stroke (Table 3) was more than twice that found from the data in NASCET, which showed a perioperative stroke risk of 5% in patients seen with nondisabling cerebral infarction.[15] This discrepancy between the NASCET data and our observations likely resulted from coding irregularities, whereby a preoperative diagnosis of a recent stroke was carried over for any subsequent hospital admissions after CEA. This observation suggests that the other parameters examined for perioperative stroke risk (Table 3) may be subject to inaccuracy on the basis of these coding irregularities.

These observations highlight the strengths and weaknesses of this large database analysis. Because of limited input field size and coding inefficiencies, the Medical Provider Analysis and Review files did not accurately capture the true incidence of common diagnoses such as hypertension and may not have accurately identified all patients seen with acute strokes or TIA. Because the observed prevalence of more serious co-morbidities such as AMI,

CHF, and DM were comparable to other series, the strength of our study stems from the analysis of short- and long-term death rates with respect to these co-morbidities and age. For patients aged 65 years and older, we found that advanced age and medical co-morbidity, particularly active coronary artery disease, CHF, and DM, were associated with an increased risk of perioperative and late death.

CLINICAL RELEVANCE
AGE AND CO-MORBIDITY
Should we perform CEA on asymptomatic patients older than 80 years? Data from ACAS do not help us address this specific question because patients older than 79 years were excluded from the study. ACAS data do imply that the therapeutic value of CEA is reduced when patients have a reduced life expectancy, particularly in women who had an inexplicably higher complication rate. On the other hand, a stroke is a condition with a much higher prevalence in older patients. A population study from Rochester, Minnesota, documented a stroke rate of 0.3% in the 55- to 64-year age group and 1.8% in those patients older than 75 years.[16] Not all these strokes are caused by carotid atherosclerosis, but undoubtedly extracranial carotid stenosis represents a major treatable cause.

Several established vascular surgery centers have reported their experience with CEA in octogenarians. O'Hara from the Cleveland Clinic group examined the early and late outcomes of CEA in 167 octogenarians.[17] Fifty-five percent had asymptomatic critical stenosis, and the overall perioperative complication rate was admirably low—the stroke rate was 2.7% and the death rate was 0.6%. Increasing age, renal insufficiency, and chronic obstructive pulmonary disease were identified as independent predictors of a decreased survival duration after operation. Most late deaths were due to cardiac disease (30%), strokes (11%), and malignancies (11%). The statistical 5-year stroke-free rate was 85%, and the 5-year survival rate was 45%.

Coyle et al.[18] from Emory University reported their results with CEA in octogenarians during a 10-year period. Seventy-nine CEAs were performed, and 44% of the patients had asymptomatic stenosis. The perioperative stroke/death rates were a remarkable 1.3% (one patient), and they documented no ipsilateral strokes in the follow-up period (mean, 35 months). Long-term follow-up was available for 80% of the patients and showed that 46% were dead by 5 years, predominantly from cardiac disease.

These investigators clearly demonstrate that CEA can be performed with low morbidity and mortality rates in experienced vascular centers. However, the follow-up data do not provide a strong basis for supporting the use of CEA in asymptomatic octogenarians. In O'Hara's study, the stroke-free rate at 5 years (85%) was less than that for the medically treated arm in ACAS (89%).[17] Furthermore, both of the aforementioned studies confirm that after 5 years about half the patients are dead, predominantly from cardiac co-morbidity. In ACAS, the survival analysis curves for the primary endpoints (i.e., an ipsilateral stroke, a perioperative stroke and death) became significant in favor of surgery after 3 years, and the annual mortality rate was 3.7% vs. 10% for the octogenarian patients.

Data from a recent study by Hsia and colleagues[19] are consistent with our observations about outcomes after CEA in Medicare patients. Death rates for patients older than 84 years were twice that of patients aged 65 to 74 years throughout the 9-year study. Campbell et al.[20] examined the outcome after CEA in a large series of patients with diabetes and found, compared with patients without diabetes, similar perioperative complication rates but dramatically reduced survival rates. After 4 years, 56% of the patients with diabetes had died compared with 25% of patients without diabetes.

These facts confirm that ACAS results cannot be extrapolated to patients older than 80 years and that the benefit of CEA is critically dependent on both the perioperative complication rate and the short-term survival rate, particularly in elderly patients. The available data suggest that octogenarians with active co-morbidities such as angina pectoris, CHF, DM, renal insufficiency, or other serious conditions do not benefit from a CEA for asymptomatic disease.

HOSPITAL AND SURGEON CASE VOLUME

Hsia and colleagues[21] from the United States Department of Health and Human Services studied the epidemiologic characteristics of CEA between 1985 and 1989 using Medicare use files from the HCFA. They found a decreasing trend in CEAs performed during their study period: the rate of CEAs per 10,000 patients declined from 20.6 in 1985 to 14.2 in 1989. During this period, the surgical mortality rate decreased from 3.0% to 2.5%, and there was an increased risk of death in older patients having surgery in low-volume hospitals. Interestingly, high-volume hospitals (i.e., greater than 75 CEAs per year) accounted for 25% of all CEAs in 1985 but only 16% in 1989. Stukenborg[22] examined hospital CEA volume in greater detail using 1989 Medicare data and found that 34% of hospitals performed 5 or less and 52% performed 10 or less CEAs that year. Only 6% of hospitals had an annual volume of CEAs more than 50.

Richardson and Main[23] documented an inverse relationship between the operating surgeon's annual case volume and the incidence of perioperative strokes among Medicare beneficiaries in Kentucky. Specifically, surgeons with annual CEA volumes less than 3 per year had a disproportionate number of major complications and a stroke rate of 6.1% vs. 2.3% for surgeons who performed more than 12 CEAs per year (Table 6). Interestingly, the majority of complications among low–case volume surgeons were attributable to only 10% of the group. In addition, they could find no correlation between the total hospital volume of CEAs and outcomes because there was significant variability in outcomes among hospitals of similar sizes. Kucey et al.[24] examined 1,280 CEAs performed at University of Toronto–affiliated hospitals and also found improved outcomes among surgeons who performed more than 12 CEAs per year.

The detailed audit of surgeons performing CEAs presented by Richardson and Main[23] underscores the importance of tracking results for individual surgeons. Unacceptably high rates of strokes

TABLE 6.

Comparison of Carotid Endarterectomy Frequency and Perioperative Complication Rate: 1989 Medicare Data From Kentucky

	Surgeons With Less Than 3 CEAs per year	Surgeons With More Than 12 CEAs per year
No. of Surgeons	47	37
No. of CEA Cases	82	504
Proportion of CEA Cases	11%	68%
Complications		
Major Complications	22	58
Proportion of Complications	27%	11%
Strokes		
Surgeons Without Stroke Complications	42	30
Surgeons With Stroke Complications	5	7
No. of Strokes	5	12
Stroke Rate	6.1%	2.3%

Abbreviation: CEA, carotid endarterectomy.
(Adapted from Richardson JD, Main KA: Carotid endarterectomy in the elderly population: A statewide experience. *J Vasc Surg* 9:65-73, 1989.)

and other complications are not necessarily related to the size of the hospital but rather to the individual surgeon, and this is supported by our data. There is also a much greater likelihood of finding a surgeon with poor outcomes among practitioners performing CEAs in low volumes. Therefore, for asymptomatic patients to achieve the optimal benefit from CEA, surgeons should be able to perform this operation with stroke/death rates are less than 3%. It is incumbent on individual surgeons and credentialing authorities within hospitals to carefully monitor CEA results so such standards can be upheld.

FUTURE PROSPECTS

The controversy revolving around intervention for asymptomatic carotid atherosclerosis may not be resolved until we can better predict the risk of neurologic sequelae in the individual patient. Traditionally, we have relied on a single parameter of atherosclerotic disease: percent luminal stenosis. However, it is apparent that there are other important factors affecting the biological features and behavior of plaque. The development of intravascular ultrasound provided a new opportunity to make detailed observations in vivo regarding plaque composition and behavior. For example, intravascular ultrasound data have confirmed that acute coronary arterial insufficiency frequently occurs after spontaneous plaque rupture[25] and that sites of plaque rupture can be predicted on the basis of morphological features.[26,27] These studies have demonstrated that the degree of luminal stenosis plays a minor role in the natural history of an atherosclerotic coronary lesion.

Although carotid atherosclerosis has not been as well characterized as coronary artery disease, the available data suggest similarities regarding plaque behavior and the lack of dependency on luminal stenosis. For example, medically treated patients in ACAS and NASCET had a comparable severity of stenosis but a widely disparate risk of strokes (2% and 13% per year, respectively).[2,6] These observations imply other factors must be more important in the development of high-risk lesions and neurologic symptoms.

However, the preoperative identification of these factors has been elusive. Weinberger et al.[28] found that large, mural-based plaques increasing in size had the highest incidence of symptomatic disease. Weinberger et al.[29] also described an increased propensity for mural plaques to rupture and develop intraplaque hemorrhages compared with discreet, nodular lesions. O'Donnell et al.[30] showed that B-mode ultrasound was more sensitive than conventional angiography for detecting plaque hemorrhaging and ulceration. In an analysis of 79 plaque specimens, they observed that hemorrhage and ulceration were significantly more common in patients with symptomatic vs. asymptomatic cerebrovascular disease (62% vs. 37%).

Other studies have refuted the utility of duplex ultrasound to correlate plaque morphological features with behavior. Hill and Donato[31] used duplex ultrasound to characterize 84 carotid plaques as predominantly calcific ($n = 34$), fibrotic with cholesterol ($n = 26$), or hemorrhagic or ulcerative ($n = 24$) on the basis of gross and histologic findings. The authors were unable to correlate plaque morphological features with lateralizing symptoms. They also observed that duplex ultrasound missed many cases of plaque hemorrhaging and ulceration and could not differentiate between lipid and blood within the vessel wall.

Although duplex ultrasound is an extremely useful technique in the diagnosis of vascular disease, it has fallen short in its capability to ascertain plaque morphologic features and composition. This is related to several factors: (1) ultrasound is operator dependent and B-mode images may be difficult to interpret by untrained personnel, (2) spatial resolution and image contrast have traditionally been inferior to CT and MRI modalities, and (3) plaque visualization is impaired by calcification.

Recent improvements in ultrasound instrumentation may overcome these limitations. Latest generation ultrasound imaging takes advantage of increased computing power and improved imaging hardware to provide extremely clear images with a spatial resolution less than 1 mm. The imaging quality now rivals or exceeds that of other modalities such as MRI or CT. Because ultrasound is the test of choice for the evaluation of carotid stenosis, enhancement of its diagnostic utility would be a useful and cost-effective strategy in an attempt to refine the indications for surgical intervention.

REFERENCES

1. Barnett HJ, Haines HJ: Carotid endarterectomy for asymptomatic stenosis. *N Engl J Med* 328:276-278, 1993.
2. Executive Committee for the Asymptomatic Carotid Atherosclerosis Study: Endarterectomy for asymptomatic carotid artery stenosis. *JAMA* 273:1421-1428, 1995.
3. Hobson RD, Weiss DG, Fields WS, et al: Efficacy of carotid endarterectomy for asymptomatic carotid stenosis. The Veterans Affairs Cooperative Study Group. *N Engl J Med* 328:221-227, 1993.
4. Moore WS, Vescera CL, Robertson JT, et al: Selection process for surgeons in the Asymptomatic Carotid Atherosclerosis Study. *Stroke* 22:1353-1357, 1991.
5. Moore WS, Barnett HJ, Beebe HG, et al: Guidelines for carotid endarterectomy. A mulitdisciplinary consensus statement from the ad hoc Committee, American Heart Association. *Stroke* 26:188-201, 1995.

6. North American Symptomatic Carotid Endarterectomy Trial Collaborators: Beneficial effect of carotid endarterectomy in symptomatic patients with high-grade carotid stenosis. *N Engl J Med* 325:445-453, 1991.

7. Golledge J, Cuming R, Beattie DK, et al: Influence of patient-related variables on the outcome of carotid endarterectomy. *J Vasc Surg* 24:120-126, 1996.

8. Akbari CM, Pomposelli FB Jr, Gibbons GW, et al: Diabetes mellitus: A risk factor for carotid endarterectomy? *J Vasc Surg* 25:1070-1075, 1997.

9. Perler BA: The impact of advanced age on the results of carotid endarterectomy: An outcome analysis. *J Am Coll Surg* 183:559-564, 1996.

10. Eagle KA, Coley CM, Newell JB, et al: Combining clinical and thallium data optimizes preoperative assessment of cardiac risk before major vascular surgery. *Ann Intern Med* 110:859-866, 1989.

11. Estes JM, Guadagnoli E, Wolf R, et al: The impact of cardiac comorbidity after carotid endarterectomy. *J Vasc Surg* 28:577-584, 1998.

12. Plecha EJ, King TA, Pitluk HC, et al: Risk assessment in patients undergoing carotid endarterectomy. *Cardiovasc Surg* 1:30-32, 1993.

13. Jencks SF, Williams DK, Kay TL: Assessing hospital-associated deaths from discharge data. The role of length of stay and comorbidities. *JAMA* 260:2240-2246, 1988.

14. Callow AD, Mackey WC: Long-term follow-up of surgically managed carotid bifurcation atherosclerosis. *Ann Surg* 210:308-316, 1989.

15. Gasecki AP, Ferguson GG, Eliasziw M, et al: Early endarterectomy for severe carotid artery stenosis after a nondisabling stroke: Results from the North American Symptomatic Carotid Endarterectomy Trial. *J Vasc Surg* 20:288-295, 1994.

16. Matsumoto N, Whisnant JP, Kurland LT, et al: Natural history of stroke in Rochester, Minnesota, 1955 through 1969: An extension of a previous study, 1945 through 1954. *Stroke* 4:20-29, 1973.

17. Coyle KA, Smith RB III, Salam AA, et al: Carotid endarterectomy in the octogenarian. *Ann Vasc Surg* 8:417-420, 1994.

18. O'Hara PJ, Hertzer NR, Mascha EJ, et al: Cartoid endarterectomy in octogenarians: Early results and late outcome. *J Vasc Surg* 27:860-869, 1998.

19. Hsia DC, Moscoe LM, Krushat WM: Epidemiology of carotid endarterectomy among Medicare beneficiaries. *Stroke* 29:346-350, 1998.

20. Campbell DR, Hoar CS, Wheelock FC: Carotid artery surgery in diabetic patients. *Arch Surg* 119:1405-1407, 1984.

21. Hsia DC, Krushat WM, Moscoe LM: Epidemiology of carotid endarterectomies among Medicare beneficiaries. *J Vasc Surg* 16:201-208, 1992.

22. Stukenborg GJ: Comparison of carotid endarterectomy outcomes from randomized controlled trials and Medicare administrative databases. *Arch Neurol* 54:826-832, 1997.

23. Richardson JD, Main KA: Carotid endarterectomy in the elderly population: A statewide experience. *J Vasc Surg* 9:65-73, 1989.

24. Kucey DS, Bowyer B, Iron K, et al: Determinants of outcome after carotid endarterectomy. *J Vasc Surg* 28:1051-1058, 1998.
25. Davies MJ, Thomas AC: Plaque fissuring: The cause of acute myocardial infarction, sudden ischaemic death, and crescendo angina [Review]. *Br Heart J* 53:363-373, 1985.
26. Lee RT, Richardson SG, Loree HM, et al: Prediction of mechanical properties of human atherosclerotic tissue by high-frequency intravascular ultrasound imaging. An in vitro study. *Arterioscler Thromb Vasc Biol* 12:1-5, 1992.
27. Cheng GC, Loree HM, Kamm RD, et al: Distribution of circumferential stress in ruptured and stable atherosclerotic lesions. A structural analysis with histopathological correlation. *Circulation* 87:1179-1187, 1993.
28. Weinberger J, Ramos L, Ambrose JA, et al: Morphologic and dynamic changes of atherosclerotic plaque at the carotid artery bifurcation: Sequential imaging by real time B-mode ultrasonography. *J Am Coll Cardiol* 12:1515-1521, 1988.
29. Weinberger J, Marks SJ, Gaul JJ, et al: Atherosclerotic plaque at the carotid artery bifurcation. Correlation of ultrasonographic imaging with morphology. *J Ultrasound Med* 6:363-366, 1987.
30. O'Donnell TF, Erdoes L, Mackey WC, et al: Correlation of B-mode ultrasound imaging and arteriography with pathologic findings at carotid endarterectomy. *Arch Surg* 120:443-449, 1985.
31. Hill SL, Donato AT: Ability of the carotid duplex scan to predict stenosis, symptoms, and plaque structure. *Surgery* 116:914-920, 1994.

CHAPTER 3

Duplex Scanning and Spectral Analysis of Carotid Artery Occlusive Disease: Improving Relevance to Clinical Practice

Brian L. Ferris, M.D.
Resident, Vascular Surgery, Division of Vascular Surgery, Department of Surgery, Oregon Health Sciences University, Portland, Oregon

Gregory L. Moneta, M.D.
Professor of Surgery, Division of Vascular Surgery, Department of Surgery, Oregon Health Sciences University, Portland, Oregon; Department of Veterans Affairs Hospital, Portland, Oregon

Contributing pathophysiologic mechanisms of internal carotid artery (ICA) atherosclerosis leading to stroke likely include regional hemodynamics, plaque composition, plaque surface characteristics, and hypercoagulability. Clinical studies evaluating the presence and severity of these potential mechanisms have established that there are statistical relationships to the incidence of strokes.[1-3] However, stratification of these risk factors for determining the benefit of carotid endarterectomy in preventing strokes has not been determined.

An additional risk factor for a stroke, the severity of ICA stenosis, has been extensively investigated with respect to the stratification of stroke risk. Results of large, multicenter, randomized trials evaluating the efficacy of carotid endarterectomy in preventing strokes have shown that the procedure benefits appropriately selected patients.[4-8] The selection criteria used in these studies were based entirely on the severity of ICA stenosis determined by contrast angiography. These criteria include 50% to 69% and 70% to 99% angiographically determined stenosis when patients were seen with symptoms of a transient ischemic attack, transient monocular blindness, or a nondisabling stroke.[4,8] Patients with 60% to 99% angiographically determined ICA stenosis without symptoms of cerebral ischemia also benefit in terms of stroke prophylaxis from a carotid endarterectomy.[5]

QUANTIFICATION OF ICA STENOSIS

Noninvasive imaging with duplex scanners is the most frequently used method for evaluation of extracranial cerebral circulation.[9] Most studies focus primarily or exclusively on the determination of the severity of cervical ICA stenosis using B-mode and color Doppler imaging in combination with Doppler waveform analysis for the accurate quantification of ICA stenosis.[9,10]

Improvements in duplex scanner technology have increased B-mode and color flow image resolution and have also enabled Doppler sample volumes to be decreased to 1 mm^3. This permits precise acquisition of spectral waveforms crucial to the determination of ICA stenosis. Measurement of color flow images of ICA lesions with electronic calipers can also be performed.[11] However, analysis of Doppler-derived spectral waveforms has shown the best clinical and research utility for the determination of the severity of ICA stenosis. Most examiners use the duplex technique for identifying potential areas of stenosis with B-mode and color flow imaging. Doppler waveform analysis is then used for the precise quantification of ICA stenosis.

Angiography determines the severity of ICA stenosis by calculating percent diameter reduction of the narrowest part of the vessel imaged in two planes. There are three methods proposed to make this calculation (Fig 1). The site of minimum lumen diameter may be compared with the estimated normal diameter of the ICA bulb or to the measured diameters of the proximal common carotid artery (CCA) or distal cervical ICA.[9,10,12-14] These latter two methods assume minimal atherosclerotic disease in the proximal CCA or distal ICA. Of these three methods, two have been used in major multicenter trials evaluating the efficacy of carotid endarterectomy to reduce the incidence of strokes. The European Carotid Surgery Trial used the estimated diameter of the carotid bulb, were it to be free of atherosclerosis, as the reference vessel in calculations of angiographically determined stenosis, whereas the North American Symptomatic Carotid Endarterectomy Trial (NASCET) and the Asymptomatic Carotid Atherosclerosis Study

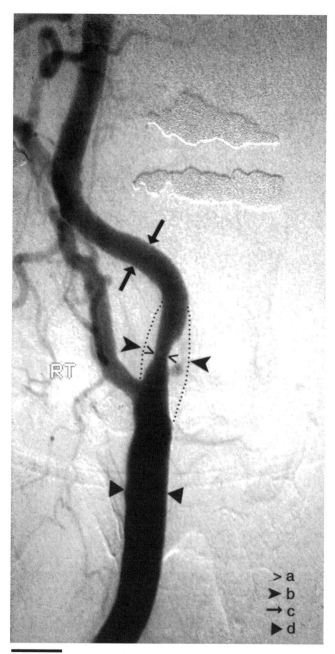

FIGURE 1.
ICA stenosis calculated using either the 1) distal ICA diameter (percent ICA stenosis=1-(a/c)*100=1-(4/7)*100=43%); 2) estimated carotid bulb diameter (percent ICA stenosis=1-(a/c)*100=1-(4/13*100=69%); or 3) common carotid artery diameter as the reference vessel (percent ICA stenosis=1-(a/c)*100=1-(4/12)*100=67%).

(ACAS) used the distal ICA as the reference vessel in calculations of angiographically determined stenosis. [6,7]

In the United States, NASCET and ACAS significantly influenced therapeutic decisions by clinicians in the treatment of carotid artery occlusive disease. NASCET initially determined that a 70% to 99% symptomatic ICA stenosis, when treated with a combination of carotid endarterectomy and medical management vs. medical management alone, resulted in a 17% absolute risk reduction for any stroke at 2 years.[4] Long-term follow-up data have shown that the protective effect is lasting; the death or disabling ipsilateral stroke rate is 6.7% at 8 years.[8] More recently, NASCET also reported that an ICA stenosis of 50% to 69% and symptoms of nondisabling cerebral ischemia can be associated with a 6.5% absolute reduction of ipsilateral strokes at 5 years by the use of carotid endarterectomy.[8] With regard to asymptomatic disease, ACAS determined that a 60% to 99% stenosis of the ICA without symptoms of cerebral ischemia, when treated by carotid endarterectomy and medical management, will have a 5.9% absolute risk reduction of ipsilateral strokes at 5 years compared with treatment with medical management alone.[5]

Both NASCET and ACAS used the distal ICA as the reference vessel to determine angiographic percent diameter reduction of the ICA. The recommendation that a carotid endarterectomy will reduce the incidence of strokes, by both NASCET and ACAS, assumes clinicians will use the distal ICA as the reference site in calculations of angiographically determined ICA stenosis.

Analyses of Doppler-derived blood flow velocity waveforms for quantification of ICA stenosis by duplex scanning are based on the comparison of duplex waveforms and carotid angiography. Fine differences in stenosis as determined by angiography cannot be delineated by duplex scanning. Relatively broad categories of stenosis as classified by duplex scanning are required for the duplex technique to be accurate.[10] Such criteria were developed by the University of Washington (UW) and are widely used both in research studies of the natural history of carotid artery stenosis and in clinical practice.

The UW criteria were developed by using the estimated normal diameter of the ICA bulb as the reference vessel in calculations of angiographically determined stenosis. The UW criteria consist of six categories of ICA stenosis (Table 1): (A) 0% stenosis (normal), (B) 1% to 15% stenosis, (C) 16% to 49% stenosis, (D) 50% to 79% stenosis, (D+) 80% to 99% stenosis, and (E) 100% stenosis (occluded).[10] The Doppler-derived spectral waveforms are acquired at an angle of insonation of 60 degrees. They are based on the determination of peak systolic velocity (PSV), end-diastolic

TABLE 1.

University of Washington Duplex Criteria to Grade Carotid Stenosis

% Stenosis Category	Velocity (cm/sec)	Spectral Characteristics
0%	PSV < 125	No spectral broadening
1% to 15%	PSV < 125	Spectral broadening in systolic deceleration
16% to 49%	PSV < 125	Spectral broadening throughout systole
50% to 79%	PSV > 125	Extensive spectral broadening
80% to 99%	PSV > 125 and EDV > 140	Extensive spectral broadening
Occluded	No flow detected	

Abbreviations: PSV, peak systolic velocity; *EDV,* end-diastolic velocity.

velocity (EDV), and the presence or absence of spectral broadening to assign a severity category. Prospective clinical studies evaluating the efficacy of this technique and the accuracy of the UW criteria have shown a sensitivity of 99%, a specificity of 85%, and an accuracy of 85% in comparison with angiography for identification and quantification of atherosclerotic occlusive disease at the carotid bifurcation.[10]

Unfortunately, the UW duplex criteria to determine the severity of ICA stenosis are not directly applicable to the results of NASCET and ACAS. First, the categories of stenosis used in the UW criteria do not directly apply to the 70% or greater threshold level of NASCET and the 60% or greater threshold level of ACAS. Second, NASCET and ACAS determined the severity of ICA stenosis using the distal ICA as the reference vessel, whereas the UW criteria determined the severity of ICA stenosis using the estimated diameter of the normal carotid bulb as the reference vessel.

Measurement of angiographically determined ICA stenosis using different vessels in the denominator (reference vessel) of calculations of stenosis has a profound effect on the calculated value of ICA stenosis. This, in turn, influences the selection of patients for carotid endarterectomy using the stenotic threshold guidelines of NASCET and ACAS. A study of 1,001 angiograms obtained from the medical arm of the European Carotid Surgery Trial found a 36% incidence of at least 70% to 99% ICA stenosis if the carotid bulb was used as the reference vessel.[12] In contrast, only 16% of the same vessels were classified as having at least 70% to 99% ICA stenosis when the distal ICA was used as the reference vessel. In addition, the variation in calculated percent stenosis using the two methods is not linear. Greater discrepancies exist when more moderate lesions are compared than when more severe stenoses are compared.[9,15] For example, proximal ICA stenosis with a 6-mm residual lumen and an estimated normal carotid bulb diameter of 12 mm has 50% stenosis when the carotid bulb is used as the reference vessel. If the distal ICA diameter is 6 mm, the calculated stenosis is 0% when the distal ICA is used as the reference vessel. In contrast, severe ICA stenosis with a 1-mm residual lumen would have 92% calculated stenosis using the carotid bulb as the reference vessel and 83% calculated stenosis using the distal ICA as the reference vessel.

SUPPLEMENTAL DUPLEX CRITERIA

These factors led us and other groups to develop supplemental duplex criteria more applicable to the results of NASCET and ACAS. These additional duplex criteria are based, once again, on the comparison of Doppler-derived spectral waveforms and carotid angiography. However, the development of these criteria applicable to NASCET and ACAS was determined using the distal ICA as the reference vessel in calculations of angiographically determined stenosis. These new criteria are not meant to replace the UW criteria, which accurately describe the severity of atherosclerosis in the carotid bulb. After all, measurements of ICA stenosis, using the distal ICA as the reference vessel, can actually be negative when the bulb is minimally diseased and maintains a larger diameter than that of the distal ICA! These new supplemental criteria are meant to assist in appropriate patient selection for carotid endarterectomy based on the results of NASCET and ACAS. Such supplemental criteria become particularly relevant when duplex scanning is the only imaging study before carotid endarterectomy. The desire to avoid preoperative angiography and to perform carotid endarterectomy based on duplex imaging alone is driven by the desire to reduce cost and to avoid the potential complications from carotid angiography. In ACAS, nearly half of the neurologic complications attributed to the surgical arm of the trial were actually complications from carotid angiography.[5] Because the therapeutic index for carotid endarterectomy, in particular asymptomatic stenosis, is quite narrow, reducing neurologic complications by minimizing cerebral angiography is crucial in maintaining the efficacy of carotid endarterectomy.

Threshold duplex criteria applicable to the results of NASCET and ACAS were initially developed at our institution. Receiver operating characteristic (ROC) curves were used to develop these criteria. ROC curves emphasize that each combination of duplex variables (PSV, EDV, ICA-PSV to CCA-PSV ratio) will have different sensitivities and specificities for predicting an angiographic threshold level of ICA stenosis based on duplex scanning.

The combination of sensitivity and specificity from any duplex variable or combination of duplex variables used to implicate the presence of a threshold level of angiographically determined ICA stenosis can be varied depending on the natural history of the disease and the risk of treatment. For example, if the natural history of a disease is poor, and the treatment is low risk and effective, a threshold value that has a very high sensitivity for identifying the disease would be chosen. The inevitable lower specificity would be accepted so that the opportunity to treat a virulent disease with a low-risk and efficacious therapy would not be missed. Treating some normal cases as a result of the lower specificity would be accepted if the treatment itself was of low risk. In contrast, if the treatment is high risk and the disease is relatively benign, one would prefer a test with a very high specificity. In such a case, the resulting lower sensitivity would be acceptable. It would be imprudent to subject any normal cases to treatment, whereas not treating some patients with the disease would be reasonable given the relatively benign nature of the disease and the relative high risk of treatment.

NASCET DUPLEX CRITERIA

Our initial study retrospectively identified threshold criteria for determining at least 70% to 99% angiographically determined ICA stenosis.[15] Carotid duplex scans obtained using Acuson duplex scanners were compared with carotid angiograms in 184 patients. Angiographically determined ICA stenosis was calculated using the distal ICA as the reference vessel, as in NASCET and ACAS. A number of variables were examined including PSV, EDV, and the ratio of ICA-PSV to CCA-PSV.

A PSV greater than or equal to 325 cm/sec and an ICA-PSV to CCA-PSV ratio of 4.0 to 4.2 were found to have the highest accuracy for determining at least 70% to 99% angiographically determined stenosis. An ICA-PSV to CCA-PSV ratio of 4 had the combination of highest sensitivity and highest accuracy in predicting at least 70% to 99% angiographically determined ICA stenosis (sensitivity, 91%; specificity, 90%; positive predictive value [PPV], 87%; negative predictive value [NPV], 94%; and accuracy, 91%). A high sensitivity was believed important as the benefit from endarterectomy in patients with 70% or greater symptomatic ICA stenosis is quite high.

The capability of an ICA to CCA/PSV ratio of 4.0 to predict at least 70% to 99% ICA stenosis was then tested in a prospective study of 168 carotid arteries using vascular laboratories in two university medical centers (Oregon Health Sciences University and the University of Washington).[16] In this study, both Acuson and Advanced Technology Laboratories (ATL) duplex scanners were used. An ICA-PSV to CCA-PSV ratio of 4.0 or greater predicted at least 70% to 99% angiographically determined ICA stenosis with a sensitivity of 90%, a specificity of 90%, a PPV of 86%, an NPV of 94%, and an accuracy of 90%. Acuson and ATL scanners provided similar velocity measurements for like degrees of ICA stenosis.

Other groups have also published supplemental duplex criteria for identification of at least 70% to 99% angiographically determined ICA stenosis using the distal ICA as the reference vessel in calculations of stenosis. These criteria and the duplex scanners used to acquire the spectral waveforms are summarized in Table 2.[17-19]

The final results of NASCET have shown that carotid endarterectomy reduces the risk of ipsilateral strokes in cases in which there is 50% to 69% ICA stenosis associated with symptoms of cerebral ischemia.[8] Duplex criteria, based on the comparison to angiography using the distal ICA as the reference vessel, have been proposed for the identification of a 50% ICA stenosis threshold. An analysis by Winkelaar et al.[20] compared the results of duplex scanning and angiography in 188 carotid arteries. An ICA-PSV to CCA-PSV ratio of 3.6 or greater was found to have a PPV of 98% for predicting more than 50% ICA stenosis. The sensitivity, however, was only 77%. Analysis of our data from 352 carotid arteries suggests that an ICA-PSV to CCA-PSV ratio of 2.7 or greater predicts 50% NASCET stenosis with an overall accuracy of 88% (sensitivity, 91%; specificity, 86%; PPV, 87%; and NPV, 90%).

TABLE 2.

Supplemental Duplex Criteria for 70% to 99% ICA Stenosis

Author	Scanner Model	Supplemental Criteria	Accuracy
Carpenter et al.	Hewlett-Packard	PSV > 210 EDV > 70 ICA-PSV:CCA-PSV > 3.0	83%
Hood et al.	Quantum	PSV > 130 EDV > 100	95%
Neale et al.	Acuson	PSV > 270 EDV > 110	93%

Abbreviations: ICA, internal carotid artery; PSV, peak systolic velocity; EDV, end-diastolic velocity; CCA, common carotid artery

ACAS DUPLEX CRITERIA

Our group also initially published duplex criteria for identifying at least 60% to 99% ICA stenosis, which is the threshold level of asymptomatic ICA stenosis determined by ACAS at which patients gain a benefit from carotid endarterectomy.[21] The benefit from a carotid endarterectomy for a patient with asymptomatic ICA stenosis, as determined by ACAS, however, is relatively modest. We therefore believe that supplemental duplex criteria for identifying patients who meet ACAS criteria should have a PPV of 95% or greater if a carotid endarterectomy were to be performed solely on the basis of duplex scanning. The resulting decrease in sensitivity provided by such a high PPV would be acceptable because of the only modest benefit of a carotid endarterectomy to reduce the risk of ipsilateral strokes in asymptomatic patients.

An analysis of 352 carotid arteries was performed using the same methods used in establishing duplex criteria for at least 70% to 99% angiographically determined ICA stenosis. ROC curves were used to identify criteria that provided a PPV of 95%. Based on this analysis, a combination of a PSV of 290 cm/sec or greater and an EDV of 80 cm/sec or greater identified 60% to 99% ICA stenosis with a PPV of 95%, a sensitivity of 78%, a specificity of 96%, and an accuracy of 88%.

Other groups have also published supplemental criteria for duplex identification of at least 60% to 99% angiographically determined ICA stenosis using the distal ICA as the reference vessel in calculations of stenosis. These results and the duplex scanners used in those studies are summarized in Table 3.[22,23]

The apparent differences between criteria proposed by our group and that of other groups were evaluated by Fillinger et al.[24] Four duplex scanners from three manufacturers in two vascular laboratories were used to produce duplex criteria for the determination of at least 60% to 99% angiographically determined ICA stenosis.

TABLE 3.

Supplemental Duplex Criteria for 60% to 99% ICA Stenosis

Author	Scanner Model	Supplemental Criteria	Accuracy
Carpenter et al.	Hewlett-Packard	PSV > 230 or EDV > 60	94% 96%
Jackson et al.	Quantum	PSV > 245 and EDV > 65	89%

Abbreviations: ICA, internal carotid artery; *PSV,* peak systolic velocity; *EDV,* end-diastolic velocity;

Each machine produced seemingly different criteria. Criteria were not interchangeable between duplex machines. Results for an ICA PSV that predicted at least 60% to 99% angiographically determined ICA stenosis with 90% or greater accuracy and a 90% or greater PPV ranged from 190 cm/sec to 240 cm/sec depending on the scanner used. Similarly, the ratio of ICA-PSV to CCA-PSV that predicted 60% to 99% angiographically determined ICA stenosis ranged from 2.6 to 3.3 depending on the scanner used.

Fillinger et al.[24] also analyzed their results using logarithmic linear regression analysis to confirm that the duplex results were, indeed, machine specific. Differences in reported duplex parameters that identify threshold levels of ICA stenosis therefore appear to be a function of differences between machines. The machines are all internally accurate based on the design properties of each machine; however, they provide different values, which makes it difficult to extrapolate data from one machine to another.

This question of variability among duplex scanners was also studied using a phantom string model by Daigle et al.[25] The accuracy of Acuson, ATL, Diasonics, and Quantum multielement linear array scanners were examined using a water-immersed string loop model at a known peak velocity of 93 cm/sec. Multiple duplex spectral waveforms were acquired using a sample volume of 1.4 mm^3 to 1.5 mm^3 at insonation angles of 50, 60, and 70 degrees. There was considerable overestimation of the phantom velocity by all scanners tested; the overestimation ranged from 5% to 15% above the string phantom velocity with the Quantum scanner to 25% to 60% above the string phantom velocity with the Acuson scanner. Some scanners were also found to have significant intraobserver variability in serial measurements of the phantom velocity. A detailed analysis showed that the accuracy was improved using measurements obtained at an insonation angle of 50 to 60 degrees. Internal quality controls are therefore required in each vascular laboratory to ensure the accuracy of carotid artery duplex scanning for that particular vascular laboratory.

BILATERAL ICA STENOSIS

Because of compensatory flow, duplex scanning may overestimate the severity of modest ICA stenosis when the contralateral side is highly stenosed or occluded. Busuttil et al.[26] reported a retrospective analysis of 550 carotid endarterectomies performed during a 7-year period. Duplex scanning overestimated the severity of ICA stenosis in 146 (26.5%) of the 550 examinations analyzed when compared with angiography.[26] Overestimation of the severity of ICA stenosis occurred in 128 (27%) of 474 ICAs that were contralateral to 80% to 99% ICA stenosis and 18 (24%) of 76 ICAs contralateral to an occlusion. After carotid endarterectomy for 80% to 99% ICA stenosis, 52% of ICAs examined decreased by one duplex category. There was an average reduction in peak systolic frequency of 11.2 MHz and an average reduction in end-diastolic frequency of 0.5 MHz.

At our institution, we reviewed 489 patients who underwent carotid endarterectomies. Preoperative duplex scanning, using the UW criteria, identified 136 patients in whom there was contralateral 50% to 99% ICA stenosis. There were 38 ICAs contralateral to the operated carotid artery that met our ACAS threshold duplex criteria, and 26 that had 80% to 99% ICA stenosis based on the UW criteria. Postoperative duplex scanning indicated that 9 (33%) of the 26 contralateral ICAs originally categorized as having 80% to 99% stenosis had changes in their Doppler waveforms postoperatively that recategorized the stenosis as 50% to 79%. The mean decrease in PSV was 46 cm/sec, and the mean decrease in EDV was 44 cm/sec for this group. Postoperative duplex scanning identified that 8 (21.1%) of the 38 contralateral ICAs categorized as ACAS candidates did not satisfy these criteria after endarterectomy of the ipsilateral ICA. The mean decrease in PSV in this group was 48 cm/sec, and the mean decrease in EDV was 36 cm/sec. These findings indicate that repeat duplex scanning is required before performing a second endarterectomy for asymptomatic disease if angiography is not performed preoperatively.

Most patients who have screening examinations for asymptomatic carotid stenosis will not have ACAS threshold lesions. To determine appropriate follow-up for patients with negative screening carotid studies, we used our duplex criteria for at least 60% to 99% ICA stenosis in a prospectively observed population of 263 patients with 434 asymptomatic duplex-derived ICA stenoses that were less than 60% to 99%.[27] Patients were examined with carotid duplex screening every 6 months and underwent an average of four examinations; the mean follow-up time was 20 months. Only 18 (4%) of 434 ICAs were found to subsequently meet our ACAS threshold criteria at repeat examination. No demographic patient or clinical criteria correlated with ICA progression to 60% to 99% ICA stenosis. An analysis of duplex spectral data, however, identified that an ICA with a PSV of more than 175 cm/sec at the time of the initial carotid screening study had a 31% incidence of progression to 60% to 99% ICA stenosis during follow-up. If the ICA PSV was less than 175 cm/sec on the initial duplex examination, only 1.8% of the ICAs progressed to at least 60% to 99% stenosis during follow-up. The life table-determined rate of freedom from progression to at least 60% to 99% angiographically determined ICA stenosis was only 14% at 3 years if the initial ICA PSV was more than 175 cm/sec. Although the follow-up period of this study was modest, the results suggest that close follow-up (perhaps every 6 months) of patients with PSVs greater than 175 cm/sec is indicated. Patients with PSVs less than 175 cm/sec likely require no more than yearly or every other year follow-up.

In conclusion, the information presented represents modifications of heretofore accepted concepts of carotid artery duplex scanning. Carotid artery duplex scanning clearly remains the best noninvasive method of assessing stenosis at the carotid bifurcation. However, despite the proven utility of carotid duplex scanning, it must be continually re-examined to ensure that it remains maximally clinically relevant with respect to current thinking on the evaluation and treatment of carotid bifurcation stenosis.

REFERENCES

1. Sitzer M, Müller W, Rademacher J, et al: Color-flow Doppler-assisted duplex imaging fails to detect ulceration in high-grade internal carotid artery stenosis. *J Vasc Surg* 23:461-465, 1996.
2. Arnold JAC, Modaresi KB, Thomas N, et al: Carotid plaque characterization by duplex scanning: Observer error may undermine current clinical trials. *Stroke* 30:61-65, 1999.
3. Golledge J, Cuming R, Ellis M, et al: Carotid plaque characteristics and presenting symptom. *Br J Surg* 84:1697-1701, 1997.
4. NASCET Collaborators: Beneficial effect of carotid endarterectomy in symptomatic patients with high grade carotid stenosis. *N Engl J Med* 325:445-453, 1991.
5. Executive Committee for ACAS: Endarterectomy for asymptomatic carotid artery stenosis. *JAMA* 273:1421-1428, 1995.
6. European Carotid Surgery Trialists' Collaborative Group: MRC European Carotid Surgery Trial: Interim results for symptomatic patients with severe (70-99%) or with mild (0-29%) carotid stenosis. *Lancet* 337:1235-1243, 1991.
7. European Carotid Surgery Trialists' Collaborative Group: Randomised trial of endarterectomy for recently symptomatic carotid stenosis: Final results of the MRC European Carotid Surgery Trial (ECST). *Lancet* 351:1379-1387, 1998.
8. Barnett HJM, Taylor DW, Eliasziw M, et al: Benefit of carotid endarterectomy in patients with symptomatic moderate or severe stenosis. *N Engl J Med* 339:1415-1425, 1998.
9. Moneta GL, Saxon RR, Taylor LM, et al: Carotid imaging before endarterectomy. *Semin Vasc Surg* 8:21-28, 1995.
10. Strandness DE: *Duplex Scanning in Vascular Disorders,* ed 2. New York, Raven Press, 1993.
11. Comerota AJ, Cranley JJ, Katz ML, et al: Real-time B- mode carotid imaging. *J Vasc Surg* 1:84-95, 1984.
12. Rothwell PM, Gibson RJ, Slattery J, et al: Equivalence of measurements of carotid stenosis: A comparison of three methods on 1001 angiograms. *Stroke* 12:2435-2439, 1994.

13. Alexandrov AV, Bladin CF, Maggisano R, et al: Measuring carotid stenosis: Time for reappraisal. *Stroke* 24:1292-1296, 1993.
14. Vanninen B, Manninen H, Koivisto J, et al: The best method to quantitate angiographic carotid artery stenosis? *Stroke* 25:708-709, 1994.
15. Moneta GL, Edwards JM, Chitwood RW, et al: Correlation of North American Symptomatic Carotid Endarterectomy Trial (NASCET) angiographic definition of 70% to 99% internal carotid artery stenosis with duplex scanning. *J Vasc Surg* 17:152-159, 1993.
16. Edwards JM, Moneta GL, Papanicolaou TG, et al: Prospective validation of new duplex ultrasound criteria for 70-99% internal carotid stenosis. *JEMU* 16:3-7, 1995.
17. Carpenter JP, Lexa FJ, Davis JT: Determination of duplex Doppler ultrasound criteria: Appropriate to the North American Symptomatic Carotid Endarterectomy Trial. *Stroke* 27:695-699, 1996.
18. Hood DB, Mattos MA, Mansour A, et al: Prospective evaluation of new duplex criteria to identify a 70% internal carotid stenosis. *J Vasc Surg* 23:254-261, 1996.
19. Neale ML, Chambers JL, Kelly AT, et al: Reappraisal of duplex criteria to assess significant carotid stenosis with special reference to reports from the North American Symptomatic Carotid Endarterectomy Trial and the European Surgery Trial. *J Vasc Surg* 20:642-649, 1994.
20. Winkelaar GB, Chen JC, Salvian AJ, et al: New duplex ultrasound criteria for managing symptomatic ≥ 50% carotid stenosis. *J Vasc Surg*, in press.
21. Moneta GL, Edwards JM, Papanicolaou G, et al: Screening for asymptomatic internal carotid artery stenosis: Duplex criteria for discriminating 60% to 99% stenosis. *J Vasc Surg* 21:989-994, 1995.
22. Carpenter JP, Lexa FJ, Davis JT: Determination of sixty percent or greater carotid artery stenosis by duplex Doppler ultrasonography. *J Vasc Surg* 22:697-705, 1995.
23. Jackson MR, Chang AS, Robles HA: Determination of 60% or greater carotid stenosis: A prospective comparison of magnetic resonance angiography and duplex ultrasound with conventional angiography. *Ann Vasc Surg* 12:236-243, 1998.
24. Fillinger MF, Baker RJ, Zwolak RM, et al: Carotid duplex criteria for a 60% or greater angiographic stenosis: Variation according to equipment. *J Vasc Surg* 24:856-864, 1996.
25. Daigle RJ, Stavros AT, Lee RM: Overestimation of velocity and frequency values by multielement linear array Dopplers. *J Vasc Technol* 14:206-213, 1990.
26. Busuttil SJ, Franklin DP, Youkey JR, et al: Carotid duplex overestimation of stenosis due to severe contralateral disease. *Am J Surg* 172:144-148, 1996.
27. Nehler MR, Moneta GL, Lee RW, et al: Improving selection of patients with less than 60% asymptomatic internal carotid artery stenosis for follow-up carotid artery duplex scanning. *J Vasc Surg* 23:580-587, 1996.

CHAPTER 4

Carotid Endarterectomy by the Eversion Technique

Dhiraj M. Shah, M.D.
Professor of Surgery, Albany Medical College, Director, Vascular
Institute, Albany Medical Center, Albany, New York

R. Clement Darling III, M.D.
Associate Professor of Surgery, Albany Medical College, Chief, Division
of Vascular Surgery, Albany Medical Center, Albany, New York

Benjamin B. Chang, M.D.
Assistant Professor of Surgery, Albany Medical College, Surgeon, Albany
Medical Center, Albany, New York

Paul B. Kreienberg, M.D.
Assistant Professor of Surgery, Albany Medical College, Surgeon, Albany
Medical Center, Albany, New York

Philip S.K. Paty, M.D.
Associate Professor of Surgery, Albany Medical College, Surgeon,
Albany Medical Center, Albany, New York

William E. Lloyd, M.D.
Assistant Professor of Surgery, Albany Medical College, Surgeon, Albany
Medical Center, Albany, New York

E version endarterectomy has a history almost as old as carotid
endarterectomy itself. An early report by DeBakey et al.[1] discussed the use of a form of eversion endarterectomy in which the
distal common carotid was transected and the plaque was
removed by everting both internal and external carotid arteries
simultaneously. Unfortunately, leaving both these arteries con-
nected minimized the operator's ability to evert and visualize the

distal end point; therefore, it was not considered reliable to remove plaque from the internal carotid artery in patients whose disease extended above the orifice. Because of this limitation, this method never reached acceptance.

For many years, eversion endarterectomy was, at best, rarely, if ever, performed for carotid disease. The most effective application of the eversion endarterectomy procedure involved its use in the external iliac and common femoral arteries, where it had been performed with excellent results.[2,3] Eversion endarterectomy of these arteries allows the surgeon to remove the plaque while directly visualizing the end point when performing a nonstenosing reconstruction. Conceptually, therefore, eversion endarterectomy can and does work as a means of autogenous arterial reconstruction.

Eversion endarterectomy for the treatment of carotid bifurcation disease was revived with a report by Kasprzak and Raithel in 1989.[4] The major and crucial difference between the original eversion endarterectomy technique and the method reported by these investigators involved the transection of the internal carotid artery at its origin at the carotid bulb. In contradistinction to the older technique, transection at this level allows for excellent visualization and, therefore, complete removal of plaque in almost all cases of carotid bifurcation atherosclerosis. The initial report was followed by several reports, generally from Europe, regarding the use of this technique. Also, some European and North American Centers have shown that eversion endarterectomy of the internal carotid artery, an alternative technique that avoids the suture line on the distal internal carotid artery, may reduce early occlusion and minimize restenosis rates.[5-8] Various surgeons, including those at our institution, tried this new technique originally in selected cases, but currently it is the preferred operation of choice for patients seen with symptomatic or asymptomatic carotid artery stenosis at our institution.

Until recently, there was almost unanimous agreement as to the general method of carotid endarterectomy: a longitudinal arteriotomy extending from the distal common carotid up on to the internal carotid artery across the area of disease was used.

Because the carotid endarterectomy technique has been performed with excellent results during the past 3 decades with minimal changes in the conventional technique, most vascular surgeons are reluctant to change. The primary advantage of eversion endarterectomy of the carotid artery is that the reanastomosis, or closure, of the arteriotomy allows for all the benefits of a conventional endarterectomy. However, the internal carotid artery reanastomosis onto the common carotid can be performed more quickly and simply with almost no chance of closure-related restenosis because the anastomosis is on the largest part of the two major vessels. There is no longitudinal or end point closure that is on the distal, and obviously smallest, part of the internal carotid artery. Secondly, management of the plaque extraction and end point management is likewise more straightforward, although cases that would be difficult to manage with conventional techniques may also be difficult with eversion. Thus, these two seemingly small advantages can relate to minimization of carotid cross-clamp time, usually on the average of 12 minutes, and minimization of the total operative time, which has been less than an hour in 85% of our procedures. This has been accomplished with an even lower rate of restenosis than previously recorded, as well as a low and acceptable rate of stroke mortality for these procedures. In the performance of a conventional carotid endarterectomy, there are two basic technical issues that need to be satisfied to successfully complete this procedure. First, the offending atherosclerotic plaque must be removed without leaving interval plaques or loose bodies within the lumen of the carotid artery. Second, the artery walls must be reapproximated without causing stenosis. This is sometimes performed by careful primary closure but is more frequently performed with the use of an autogenous or prosthetic patch.[9-11] The use of either type of closure is associated with a low but finite frequency of stenosis either early or late in the postoperative period. Use of autogenous material often requires the use of a saphenous vein patch, and, therefore, a second operative field; use of a prosthetic patch introduces a foreign body into the wound, and some prosthetic materials may also allow troublesome bleeding at the time of the operation. Failure to successfully negotiate these technical hurdles may result in stenosis, occlusion, and, at worst, a stroke. These complications occur in a small but not inconsequential number of patients. Thus, although conventional carotid endarterectomies are familiar and time tested, they should not necessarily be automatically regarded as the last word in carotid reconstruction. There is always room for improvement in an apparently perfect system. Meticulous closure is especially important in the prevention of restenosis. Symptomatic or asymptomatic restenosis rates after carotid endarterectomy range from 2% to 30% as previously noted.[12-14] The performance of patch angioplasty closure suggests that the use of a patch minimizes restenosis. On the other hand, primary closure with a fine-suture technique in a larger artery should also result in minimal rates of restenosis. However, closure of the arteriotomy by any of these procedures, in reality, may decrease the distal diameter of the internal carotid artery. Alternatively, carotid endarterectomy by the eversion technique completely avoids the need for sutures in the distal internal carotid artery by displacing the suture line to a more proximal and much larger junction of the distal common carotid and proximal internal carotid arteries. A closure of this nature is not only technically much easier than either primary closure or patch angioplasty of the conventional longitudinal arteriotomy, but also minimizes the role of closure in restenosis.[15] Also, when the internal carotid artery is reanastomosed to the common carotid artery, usually by use of a continuous suture, the suture line of the carotid artery is at the widest part of the system, the bulb, and the distal internal carotid artery diameter usually increases rather than decreases after this procedure. In this chapter, we report the details of eversion endarterectomy—the technique, its variations, and limitations—as well as our experience and results to date.

METHODS
SELECTION OF CASES
Surgeons adopting eversion endarterectomy need not change the majority of their technique. The anesthetic choice and method of cerebral monitoring and protection can be the same for both eversion and traditional carotid endarterectomy. However, in this series, the vast majority of patients underwent carotid endarterectomy by the eversion technique under cervical block anesthesia. Shunts were only used for patients who had neurologic deterioration after carotid cross clamping.

As currently conceived, eversion endarterectomy can be used to treat almost all cases of primary carotid bifurcation disease and highly selective cases of recurrent stenosis. This technique is ideal for treatment of carotid arteries that are redundant with kinks or loops, as shortening of the artery can be more easily accomplished by this technique than by conventional methods. A common concern about eversion endarterectomy is that a shunt (either elective or routine) cannot be used. Actually, the use of a shunt, in some cases, can facilitate the completion of the procedure. Once the shunt is inserted, the internal carotid artery can be everted over this and used as a mandrel to fully remove the disease and evaluate the end point. However, certain types of shunts are probably more easily used with eversion than others, and the specifics of shunt use will be detailed later in this chapter. The extent of disease at the bifurcation may affect one's ease in performing carotid endarterectomy by any method. Disease limited to or near the bifurcation is much easier to treat than disease that travels up the internal carotid artery. Treatment of more extensive disease, for instance, disease that travels to the level of the digastric muscle, is more difficult to manage with any technique. These cases are not good cases to use when learning how to perform an eversion endarterectomy, but, with additional experience, the surgeon may be able to manage them with this technique. It is important after the initial dissection and isolation of the carotid artery to evaluate the extent of the disease, because the decision about what type of endarterectomy to perform may be based on this evaluation. If one sees yellow atheromatous plaque that can be visualized from external observation and if this melds into a purplish robin's-egg blue normal artery or does so distally, one can be relatively confident that the plaque will end and feather out nicely and that an eversion endarterectomy can be successfully and expeditiously performed. If one does not see this transition zone and the plaque extends concentrically up to the digastric muscle, then alternative methods of reconstruction should be considered.

As mentioned before, eversion endarterectomy can be used in the treatment of some recurrent lesions but is contraindicated in the treatment of others. When the original endarterectomy is performed with conventional techniques and a prosthetic patch, eversion is not appropriate for treatment of a recurrent lesion. Carotids patched with autogenous vein material may sometimes be operated on using the eversion technique, but these operations may not be universally successful. Early or late recurrent lesions may be removed by eversion, but the long-term results of this technique remain to be defined.

PERIOPERATIVE MANAGEMENT

The preoperative workup of the patient seen with carotid bifurcation disease is similar for both the eversion and the traditional endarterectomy techniques. All patients with possible carotid artery disease are evaluated clinically and with duplex scanning. If indicated, contrast angiography or MR arteriography further delineate the lesions. Preoperatively, the patient's perioperative risk for surgery is also assessed, and special attention is paid to cardiac co-morbid conditions. Occasionally, a cardiac stress test is done, followed by cardiac catheterization as indicated. Postoperatively, patients remain in the postanesthesia care unit for 2 to 4 hours until their blood pressure and neurologic status are assessed and are stable, then they are transferred to a bed in a nonintensive care unit located on a vascular floor. Usually, patients can be discharged within 24 hours of surgery. Patients who are seen with synchronous bilateral critical stenoses undergo contralateral carotid endarterectomy within the first or second postoperative day if there are no complications from the first operation, such as headaches, hypertension, hoarseness, vocal cord dysfunction, or other neurologic concerns. On discharge, patients are usually visited by home care nurses who monitor their blood pressure and look for the presence of severe headaches or wound problems. These patients will only occasionally require further intervention by physicians. After the initial 2-week postoperative visit, patients are followed-up by duplex examination of both carotid arteries at 3 months, 6 months, and once a year thereafter.

Early in our experience with eversion endarterectomy, ultrasound was performed at 3 months for the entire first year and then every 6 months thereafter for a period of 3 years. During follow-up, any complication, whether it was stenosis, occlusion, or a neurologic symptom, was prospectively recorded in our vascular registry. Reevaluation was performed for the patients in whom carotid restenosis was greater than 60% by duplex or for those who became symptomatic. Further evaluation was carried out by either MR angiography or conventional angiography as indicated.

TECHNIQUE

As previously mentioned, various techniques for eversion endarterectomy have been attempted. DeBakey et al.[1] divided the common carotid artery and performed the eversion endarterectomy of both the internal and external carotid arteries. This technique works well only for lesions that do not extend up into the internal carotid artery, as the attached external carotid artery limits the length of the internal carotid artery that may be everted. This technique was further modified by using two revisions: one on the common carotid artery and a separate transverse incision on the internal carotid artery to maximize visualization and tacking of the end point. However, most of these modifications made the procedure more complicated and technically more difficult. The basic principle of our technique simply involves the complete division of the internal carotid artery from the common carotid artery in an oblique fashion at the area of the bulb that encompasses most of the atherosclerotic disease. The line of transection may be beveled on the common carotid artery a variable distance,[4AQ] depending on the approximate extent of disease; after the internal carotid artery is divided, it is mobilized beyond the disease and the eversion is performed.[16] The many variations of our technique of eversion endarterectomy will be elucidated further in the next section.

After the patient is brought into the operating room, the neck is slightly tilted away from the affected side and a regional block anesthesia is performed by rami block from C2 to C4 supplemented by superficial infiltration of the anesthetic agent. Usually, the arterial line is inserted for blood pressure monitoring during the procedure; because the patient is awake, no EEG[5AQ] monitoring is done. A small IV bag attached to a pressure transducer is placed in the patient's contralateral hand; this bag is squeezed intermittently by the patient to monitor motor function, the ability to follow commands, and other aspects of neurologic function during and after clamping.

The initial exposure of the carotid artery is identical with either method of endarterectomy. After the anterior surface of the carotid artery is exposed, heparin may be administered. Carotid sinus nerves are usually infiltrated with 1% lidocaine to block a vagal effect. Although circumferential dissection of the internal carotid along its length is a necessary part of eversion endarterectomy, this is probably best completed after clamping and division of the artery. Thus, only sufficient dissection to effect clamping need be performed initially. After the carotid artery is exposed, the patient is given 30 U/kg body weight of IV heparin (2,000-3,000 U total). Heparin is not received after the procedure.

After clamping, the internal carotid artery is divided obliquely from the carotid bulb (Fig 1). The actual angle of transection is not precisely important but should be in the range of 30 to 60 degrees from the horizontal. It is relatively important for the line of transection to end in the crotch of the carotid bulb and not up in the internal or external carotids; failure to do so is not catastrophic but can make reanastomosis more complicated than necessary.

After the internal carotid is divided, upwards and lateral traction on the artery will help the operator see the remaining tissue adherent to the artery. This consists of the carotid sinus tissue

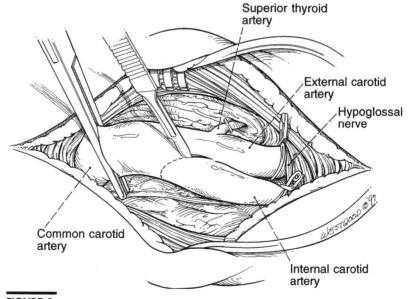

FIGURE 1.
Transsection of internal carotid artery. Copyright 1997, Wm. B. Westwood.

medially and the looser areolar tissue adherent posteriorly in which the vagus nerve usually lies. Dissection along the divided artery close to it mobilizes the remaining length of artery while avoiding injury to the surrounding structures.

At this point, the divided carotid may be externally examined. The end of the plaque may be seen as the transition from the yellowish diseased artery to the normal bluish artery. The clamp should be placed across the normal artery, ideally well above the transition zone, as this will make eversion of the artery and examination of the end point in detail easier. If a more cephalad exposure is needed, the usual measures of division of the ansa, mobilization of the hypoglossal nerve, and division of the digastric muscle may be performed. If the disease still runs superior to this point, an endarterectomy will be difficult by any technique, and the operator should use whatever method is more familiar.

After the divided carotid is fully mobilized, it usually is redundant in relation to the common carotid artery. This redundancy may range from a very few millimeters to several centimeters in those cases seen with carotid kinks or loops (Fig 2). The side of the internal carotid artery formerly adherent to the carotid body is then divided longitudinally such that the end of this arteriotomy lines up with the upper end of the common carotid arteriotomy. Also, the common carotid opening is extended caudally to match. The resultant opening in the carotid artery is usually 15 to 30 mm

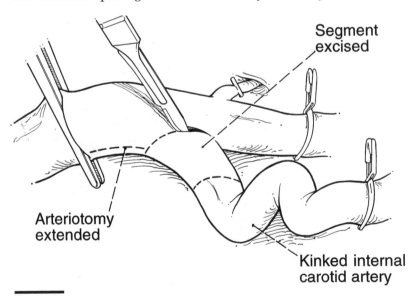

Segment excised

Arteriotomy extended

Kinked internal carotid artery

FIGURE 2.
Excision of redundant internal carotid artery. Copyright 1997. Wm. B. Westwood.

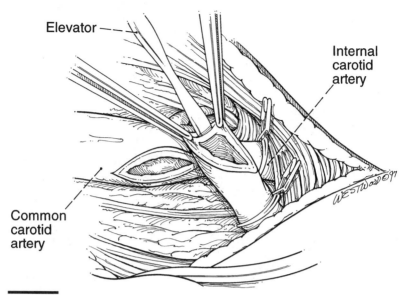

FIGURE 3.
Elevation of internal carotid plaque. Copyright 1997, Wm. B. Westwood.

in length; this is important, as the extra length will allow for a wide, easily performed anastomosis with little chance for stenosis. If the internal carotid redundancy is too much, the end could be excised and tailored to match the common carotid stoma.

At this point, if the arteriotomy goes across the end point of the plaque, a shunt may be inserted if desired. This will be elaborated on later.

Removal of the bulk of the internal carotid plaque is a simple maneuver that usually takes a few seconds. The plaque is elevated from the adventitia circumferentially (Fig 3). Care should be taken to try to include the outer layer of media with the specimen; if this is not done, the outer arterial wall will be relatively stiff and, therefore, difficult to evert. After the plane of dissection is established, one pair of forceps is used to grasp the plaque and another forceps is used to grasp the adventitia. The adventitia is then everted to the end of the plaque. Exposure is better if the adventitia is actually turned inside out as if one was peeling a banana or rolling up a sleeve (Fig 4). The forceps holding the plaque should be held in place, and the other forceps should be moved cephalad. If the plaque is merely pulled out of the artery without eversion, the end point will often be poorly visualized. If the adventitia is merely pushed cephalad and not everted, the redundant adventitia will obstruct the view of the end point.

As the end point is reached, the bulk of the plaque usually spontaneously snaps off relatively cleanly. Alternatively, the

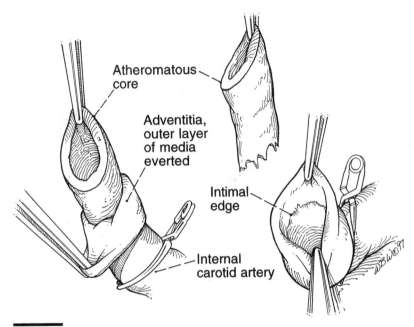

FIGURE 4.
Removal of plaque and visualization of end point. Copyright 1997, Wm. B. Westwood.

plaque may be sharply divided with either fine scissors or a no. 11 or no. 15 scalpel blade. Although these steps may seem complicated, they usually take the experienced operator 30 seconds from the division of the artery to the removal of the plaque. If a shunt was not inserted previously, it may be inserted at this time.

If the artery is fully everted, the end point is circumferentially visible at the end of the everted artery. Loose pieces of media and intima are picked or shaved off the wall. The superior visualization of the end point before closure of the artery is one of the advantages of this technique as compared with a conventional endarterectomy. Obviously, this is the most critical step of the procedure, and the operator should take the time to make the end point as perfect as possible. Sometimes, gentle irrigation of the end point will cause loose strands of tissue to float away from the adventitia such that they can be visualized and removed.

If the end point is not well visualized, the operator should make sure the artery is maximally everted. If necessary, the clamp should be moved further cephalad. Sometimes, if a bulky clamp is used, eversion is obstructed. Small clamps such as Yasargils are ideal.

If the end point is now satisfactory, the artery may be irrigated with heparinized saline. If there are still loose flaps, tacking sutures can be used. Although there are several ways to put in these types of sutures depending on the relationship of the end of the arteriotomy to the end point, the most reliable method requires the assistant to hold the bulk of the everted adventitia at two points. It often helps if the adventitia is rolled or crumpled together. The operator can then pass both needles of a double-armed suture from within the lumen to the exterior of the artery while forming a vertical mattress suture. The tacking sutures are more difficult to place when several centimeters of internal carotid need to be everted to expose the end point.

With the end point now secured with or without tacking sutures, the internal carotid is unrolled. Remaining shreds of media are removed, and the artery is irrigated. The unrolled artery is held up to the arteriotomy in the common carotid artery. The cephalad ends of both arteriotomies should be lined up and opposed. If the internal carotid is excessively redundant, the proximal end may be amputated. Otherwise, the common carotid arteriotomy is extended proximally such that the end of this arteriotomy can oppose the proximal end of the endarterectomized internal carotid artery. The two arteriotomies are both typically 15 to 30 mm long at this time.

Endarterectomy of the common carotid is done at this time and is essentially performed in the same fashion as a conventional endarterectomy (Fig 5). The plaque is elevated from the adventitia. This is continued around the entire circumference of the common carotid. Once this is completed, it is useful to transversely divide the plaque, thereby allowing the surgeon to deal with the common carotid and external carotid plaque as separate issues.

If endarterectomy of the external carotid artery is necessary or desired, the plaque is circumferentially mobilized and grasped firmly. The plaque may be extracted by a combination of traction on the plaque and partial eversion of the external carotid adventitia.

Endarterectomy of the common carotid artery can usually be simply performed by grasping the elevated plaque and amputating it from the adventitia. In cases in which the common carotid plaque runs proximally, a combination of two techniques is helpful. If the plaque extends proximal to the end of the arteriotomy no more than 2 to 3 cm, the plaque may be grasped and the common carotid artery may be everted to expose the line of transection of the plaque. Often this maneuver may be facilitated by further circumferential mobilization of the common carotid artery externally and, if necessary, by moving the clamp more caudad.

If the plaque runs so proximally that it cannot adequately be extracted by everting the common carotid artery, the arteriotomy may simply be extended proximally until the plaque diminishes. The atherosclerotic lesion may be removed by direct endarterecto-

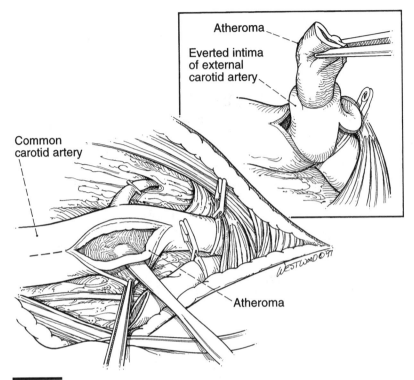

Common
carotid artery

Atheroma

Atheroma

Everted intima
of external
carotid artery

FIGURE 5.
Endarterectomy of external and common carotid arteries. Copyright 1997,
Wm. B. Westwood.

my. Closure of the additional arteriotomy may usually be performed primarily, as this artery is relatively large. This will result
in a Y-shaped suture line where the linear common carotid closure
meets the proximal suture line connecting the distal common to
the internal carotid artery. Although some operators have voiced
reluctance to reconstruct the artery in this fashion, we have done
this in more than 100 cases with no short- or long-term problems.

After the common and external carotids are adequately
endarterectomized, they are irrigated, and any residual loose fragments are removed. A fine monofilament nonabsorbable suture
(6-0 is usually ideal) is used to reanastomose the internal to the
distal common carotid artery. The suture is usually started at the
most cephalad ends of both arteriotomies, and the two mends are
brought around as desired (Fig 6). The major advantage of eversion
endarterectomy is that the arteriotomies are both 15 to 30 millimeters long and the lumens of both opened arteries are used to
"patch" each other. It is now extremely easy to sew the arteries
together without producing a stenosis. Also, the closure is done in

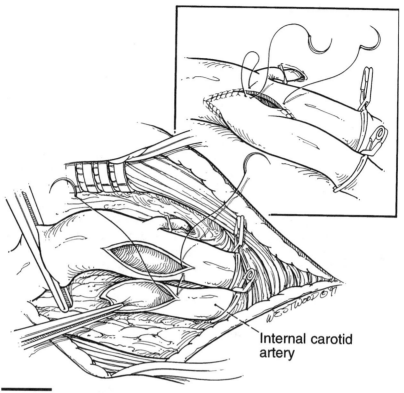

Internal carotid
artery

FIGURE 6.
Reanastomosis of internal to common carotid artery. Copyright 1997, Wm.
B. Westwood.

the more accessible center of the wound, not in the upper reach.
Conversely, it is very difficult to cause a stenosis during closure as
long as the initial three bites in the wall of the internal carotid
artery are not absurdly large. The clamps may be flashed, and the
lumen may be irrigated before the suture line is completed. After
completion, flow is instituted into the external carotid before
unclamping the internal carotid. With all arteries unclamped, the
flow is assessed by Doppler ultrasound, and the patients are
observed for neurologic changes (cervical block cases). Wounds
are closed, and drains are used as desired by the operator.

Because one of the major technical issues of carotid endarterectomy is removed by simplifying the closure, eversion endarterectomy
obviates the need for patching or tedious primary closure of the distal internal carotid artery. Removal of the plaque and establishing the
end point are also usually simpler. This simplification in technique
may be translated into a speedier operation with less stress for the
surgeon.

USE OF A SHUNT

Probably the most frequent objection or supposed contraindication to eversion endarterectomy raised by surgeons (some of whom use eversion endarterectomy) is that the use of a shunt is difficult or impossible. This is patently false. Although we usually use shunts on demand (monitored by patient responsiveness during awake anesthesia), the use of a shunt routinely or occasionally can be easily incorporated into the routine use of eversion endarterectomy.

Certain shunts do work better than others with eversion. Those shunts that are fixated at either end with either an internal balloon (Pruitt-Inahara type) or with external clamping (Javid type) are both eminently suitable for eversion techniques and may actually make eversion of the distal internal carotid easier. Unfortunately, straight shunts (Edwards type) may not be easily usable because the traction on the arteries as they are everted tends to make these shunts slip out.

Shunt insertion may be accomplished in the following fashion. After the internal carotid is divided from the common carotid and mobilized, the arteriotomy is extended cephalad a variable distance. In some cases, this extension goes through the end point, and normal lumen is visible. A shunt can be inserted at this time (Fig 7). If the end point of the plaque is not encompassed by the

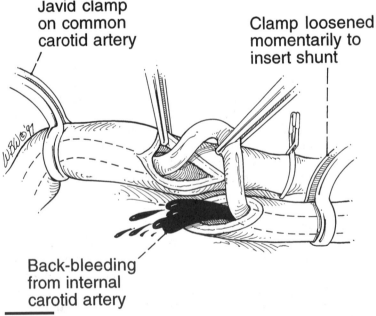

Javid clamp
on common
carotid artery

Clamp loosened
momentarily to
insert shunt

Back-bleeding
from internal
carotid artery

FIGURE 7.
Insertion of shunt past divided plaque. Copyright 1997, Wm. B. Westwood.

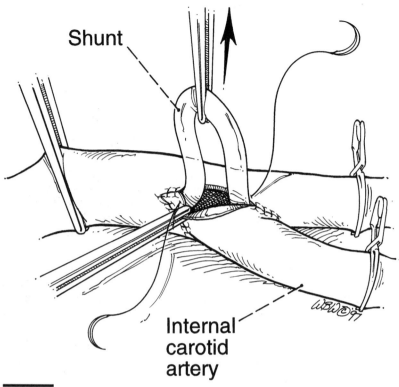

FIGURE 8.
Reanastomosis with shunt in place. Copyright 1997, Wm. B. Westwood.

arteriotomy, the bulk of the plaque is quickly everted and removed to expose the normal lumen. Shunt insertion may be performed at this time. Although the second method may seem time-consuming, usually shunt insertion may be accomplished in less than a minute after initial clamping of the arteries.

Proximal insertion of a shunt is facilitated by the usual caudad extension of the common carotid arteriotomy. This allows the surgeon to see a relatively clean artery in which to place the shunt.

After flow is instituted in the shunt, the internal carotid is everted over the shunt. If the clamp is placed cephalad enough, the shunt acts as a mandrel over which the artery is everted. This allows for unparalleled visualization of the end point.

Endarterectomy of the common carotid is completed in the standard fashion, and the shunt is put in place by the methods previously described. Reanastomosis is accomplished by completing as much of the suture line as possible while leaving the shunt protruding from the anterior surface (Fig 8). The shunt is then removed, the arteries are reclamped, and the suture line is completed in the standard fashion.

NONREDUNDANT CAROTIDS

Almost all internal carotids prove to be redundant after division and mobilization. This is the critical fact that allows the operator to extend the arteriotomy several millimeters to produce a large, easily performed reanastomosis that is one of the key advantages of the eversion technique. Infrequently, the internal carotid is not redundant after division, even with circumferential mobilization. There are generally two methods to deal with this situation.

The most straightforward technique would be to complete the endarterectomy without extending the internal and common carotid endarterectomies. Although there is nothing specifically wrong with this approach, eversion is often more difficult, especially if the plaque runs cephalad for any distance. Even more importantly, significant amounts of diseased common carotid will be difficult to extract through the 5- to 10-mm arteriotomy. Finally, shunt insertion will be difficult to impossible in many cases as the proximal plaque will prevent insertion of the larger end of the shunt.

The second general method of dealing with short internal carotid arteries addresses their limitations and uses a modification of a technique originally developed for use in a conventional endarterectomy called advancement bifurcationplasty.[17] In this method, identical arteriotomies are made in the opposed surfaces of both the internal and external carotid arteries. This obviously requires additional mobilization of the external carotid and individual control of many of its branches. After sufficient external carotid is mobilized, the arteriotomies are lengthened in a cephalad direction with care being taken to make them the same length and to orient them such that they can later be joined without twisting. This will usually leave a 15- to 30-mm arteriotomy that can easily be closed without stenosis. Opening both arteries makes extraction of the plaque easy and improves visualization of the end points. In addition, shunt insertion can be performed as previously described through the larger arteriotomies, although the common carotid plaque may still need to be debulked before insertion of the shunt.

TECHNICAL SUGGESTIONS

The adoption of any significant modification in technique is often unsettling, especially when the conventional technique seems to provide adequate results. Although eversion endarterectomy can be used effectively in all cases of primary carotid bifurcation disease, there is a certain amount of learning and experience that must be undergone before reaching this point.

The most significant issue with any endarterectomy is proper management of the end point. Although we find end point management to be easier in most cases with eversion, during the learning period, the surgeon may feel unsure about the status of the end point in some cases. There are two general methods of dealing with this problem. (The need for these maneuvers will rapidly decrease with greater operative experience with the eversion technique.)

The first method requires the operator to finish the rest of the endarterectomy, as previously described, and to reanastomose the internal to the common carotid artery. However, the arteries are left clamped, and a short vertical arteriotomy is made over the end point. The end point may be examined, flaps may be removed, and tacking sutures may be inserted by conventional techniques. The arteriotomy can then be closed with a small patch of autogenous vein or prosthetic material if desired.

The second method involves amputating the proximal internal carotid distal to the end point and performing a common carotid–internal carotid bypass. This solves the problem of a difficult end point by anchoring the entire circumference of the distal intima with a suture line. This makes the entire operation considerably more tedious and should only be used when necessary. The choice of conduit material should be either polytetrafluoroethylene or autogenous vein. Both produce similar results when used in this position, and the restenosis rate is 5% to 10%. The size of the internal carotid may often dictate the type of graft used; that is, smaller carotids are more easily size-matched with vein material, whereas it is more convenient to use polytetrafluoroethylene for the larger carotids.

We have had to apply these techniques in less than 0.5% of cases; most of these were performed in the first year of adopting the eversion technique. The techniques are rarely necessary with experience.

CLINICAL MATERIALS AND RESULTS

Eversion endarterectomy was introduced into our institution in 1993. As with any significantly new technique, there was a transition period lasting approximately 1 year during which the individual surgeons tried this method in some cases. Interestingly, all surgeons adopted this new technique as their primary method of carotid endarterectomy (Table 1). Since 1993, 2,869 carotid end-

---

TABLE 1.

Changing Technique of Carotid Endarterectomy

	1993	1994	1995	1996	1997	1998
Total CEAs	189	352	650	721	742	754
Eversion CEAs	36	130	545	692	731	739
Standard CEAs	153	222	105	29	11	15

Abbreviation: CEA, carotid endarterectomy.

TABLE 2.
Indications for Eversion Carotid Endarterectomy

	All CEAs	CEAs With CABG
Transient Ischemic Attack	409 (14.3%)	17 (4.7%)
Amaurosis Fugax	276 (9.6%)	7 (1.9%)
Stroke	245 (8.5%)	10 (2.7%)
Asymptomatic Stenosis	1,939 (67.6%)	330 (90.7%)

Abbreviations: CEA, carotid endarterectomy; *CABG,* coronary artery bypass grafting.

arterectomies have been performed using the eversion technique. The indications for the operations were symptomatic disease in 930 (32.4%) and significant asymptomatic stenosis in 1,939 (67.6%) (Table 2). Patients were predominantly men with the usual risk factors (Table 3).

Regional anesthesia was used preferentially and amounted to 2,424 cases (84.5%). There were 435 procedures performed under general anesthesia, and this choice was made because of a simultaneous coronary artery bypass grafting in 364 cases. The remaining cases were managed with general anesthesia because of surgeon or patient preference, psychiatric reasons, or inadequate regional anesthesia (Table 4).

Shunts were placed for neurologic deterioration in the cervical block cases and amounted to 4.0% (96/2,424) of the total. Shunts placed in the general anesthesia cases were somewhat more frequent (1.8%; 8/445) and driven by surgeon preference, an indication for surgery (e.g., acute strokes or crescendo transient ischemic attacks), or poor internal carotid back pressure.

TABLE 3.
Demographics

Total Procedures	2,869
Total Patients	2,358
Males	1,335 (56.6%)
Females	1,023 (43.4%)
Diabetes	582 (24.7%)
Smoking	762 (32.3%)
Hypertension	1,344 (57.0%)
Coronary Artery Disease	1,132 (48.0%)
Mean Age	70
Age Range	30-95

TABLE 4.

Operative Parameters

	All CEAs	CEAs With CABG
Anesthesia		
Block	2,424 (84.5%)	0 (0.0%)
General	435 (15.2%)	364 (100.0%)
Block to General	10 (0.3%)	0 (0.0%)
Patch	26 (0.9%)	1 (0.3%)
Shunt	103 (3.6%)	0 (0.0%)

Abbreviations: CEA, carotid endarterectomy; *CABG*, coronary artery bypass grafting.

Major postoperative complications from the 2,869 eversion endarterectomies included 23 cases of strokes and 28 cases of other major morbidities and death from nonneurologic causes. In addition, there was a low rate of other minor complications including hematomas requiring drainage (1.4%), cranial nerve injuries (0.2%), and asymptomatic early occlusion (0.2%). Of the 2,033 patients operated on only for carotid disease, 32 (1.6%) died or had strokes. The rate of these complications in the coronary artery bypass grafting–carotid group was somewhat higher (16/325 or 4.9%) (Table 5).

Follow-up included initial duplex ultrasound at our institution in all cases followed by serial duplex scans at 6- to 12-month inter-

TABLE 5.

Results

	All CEAs	CEAs With CABG
Operative Mortality	28/2,358 (1.2%)	11/325 (3.4%)
Complications		
Transient Neurologic Deficit	22 (0.8%)	
Permanent Neurologic Deficit	23 (0.8%)	
Nonfatal Cardiac	25 (0.9%)	
Nerve Injury	7 (0.2%)	
Wound Infection	3 (0.1%)	
Intracerebral Bleeding	5 (0.2%)	
Bleeding	39 (1.4%)	
Restenosis (long term)	20 (0.7%)	
Occlusion	19 (0.7%)	

Abbreviations: CEA, carotid endarterectomy; *CABG*, coronary artery bypass grafting.

TABLE 6.
Cumulative Patency and Patient Survival Rates

	Number of Months					
	1	**12**	**24**	**36**	**48**	**60**
Cumulative Patency	99.5%	99.0%	97.9%	97.9%	97.9%	97.9%
Cumulative Survival	98.7%	96.8%	92.9%	89.5%	84.5%	84.5%

vals. Interestingly, the restenosis rate was relatively low (0.7%). It has been suggested by this group and others that use of this technique may be associated with a lower rate of restenosis, possibly because there is no suture line in the region of the distal end point. The long-term patency rates of eversion endarterectomy and stroke-free survival rates were excellent (Table 6).

CONCLUSION

Carotid endarterectomy by the eversion technique has proven to be a technique that encompasses the entire scope of normal carotid surgeries. Although it is uniquely useful for the treatment of redundant internal carotid arteries, it can be used for almost all routine carotid endarterectomies. The major advantage of this technique is that the closure of the artery is no longer a major technical problem. Instead, by using the arteries to patch each other, there is little danger of producing a significant stenosis from the closure, and no extra vein or prosthetic material is needed. As elaborated in this chapter, the eversion technique may be routinely used with or without shunts.

This last point is further evidence for the fact that many surgeons believe that female patients undergoing carotid endarterectomies are more likely to require patch closure or have a higher rate of restenosis in long-term follow-up. Using the eversion technique, not only can one perform an endarterectomy on a smaller vessel that will not require a distal suture line on the internal carotid artery but also one can perform the closure of the arteriotomy without a patch, in essence using the internal to patch over the common carotid artery. Our results with this technique demonstrate a recurrence rate in women that is less than 1%, which is identical to their male cohorts.

Management of the end point requires the surgeon to learn how to evert the internal carotid artery. This is not technically difficult and requires a minimum of effort to learn. In many cases, visualization of the end point is superior to standard techniques, thereby simplifying the other major technical issue facing the operative surgeon. However, internal carotid arteries with long-running plaques will be difficult to manage no matter what technique is used. We discourage indirect visualization of the end point via angioscopy in favor of direct visualization and complete removal of the plaque.

Although it is always difficult to improve on a well-accepted technique, we believe that eversion endarterectomy is truly an advance in carotid surgery and one that we have adopted enthusiastically. We hope that other surgeons try this technique because we believe that, with a little experience, they will be equally positive about the advantages eversion endarterectomy offers. Whether this becomes the principal technique or merely an occasional technique of the operator, it is an important and useful tool for the surgeon who performs carotid procedures.

REFERENCES

1. DeBakey ME, Crawford ES, Cooley DA, et al: Surgical considerations of occlusive disease of innominate, carotid, subclavian and vertebral arteries. *Ann Surg* 149:690-710, 1959.
2. Darling RC III, Leather RP, Chang BB, et al: Is the iliac artery a suitable inflow conduit for iliofemoral occlusive disease? An analysis of 514 aortoiliac reconstructions. *J Vasc Surg* 17:15-19, 1993.
3. Inhara T: Eversion endarterectomy for aortoiliofemoral occlusive disease: A 16-year experience. *Am J Surg* 138:196-204, 1979.
4. Kasprzak PM, Raithel D: Eversion carotid endarterectomy-technique and early results. *J Cardiovasc Surg (Torino)* 30:495, 1989.
5. Berguer R: Eversion endarterectomy of the carotid bifurcation, in Veith FJ (ed): *Current Critical Problems in Vascular Surgery*, vol. 5. St Louis, Quality Medical Publishing, 1993, pp 441-447.
6. Kieny R, Hirsch D, Seiller C, et al: Does carotid eversion endarterectomy and reimplantation reduce the risk of restenosis? *Ann Vasc Surg* 7(5)407-413, 1993.
7. Koskas F, Kieffer E, Bahnini A: Carotid eversion endarterectomy: Short- and long-term results. *Ann Vasc Surg* 9:9-15, 1995.
8. Reigner B, Reveilleau P, Gayral M, et al: Eversion endarterectomy of the internal carotid artery: Mid-term results of a new technique. *Ann Vasc Surg* 9:141-146, 1995.
9. AbuRhama AF, Khan JH, Robinson PA, et al: Prospective randomized trial of carotid endarterectomy with primary closure and patch angioplasty with saphenous vein, jugular vein, and polytetrafluoroethylene: Perioperative (30-day) results. *J Vasc Surg* 24:998-1007, 1996.
10. Counsell CE, Salinas R, Naylor R, et al: A systematic review of the randomized trials of carotid patch angioplasty in carotid endarterectomy. *Eur J Vasc Endovasc Surg* 13:345-354, 1997.
11. Eikelboom BC: Carotid endarterectomy: Patch versus primary closure, in Bernstein EF, Callow AB, Nicolaides AN, et al (eds): *Cerebral Revascularization*. London, Med-Orion, 1993, pp 309-315.

12. Chervu A: Recurrent carotid artery stenosis: Diagnosis, management, and prevention. *Semin Vasc Surg* 8:70-76, 1995.
13. Das MB, Hertzer NR, Ratliff NB, et al: Recurrent carotid stenosis: A five-year series of 65 reports. *Ann Surg* 202:28-35, 1985.
14. Zierler RE, Bandyk DF, Thiele BL, et al: Carotid artery stenosis following endarterectomy. *Arch Surg* 117:1408-1415, 1982.
15. Cao P, Giordano G, DeRango P, et al: A randomized study on eversion versus standard carotid endarterectomy: Study design and preliminary results: The Everest Trial. *J Vasc Surg* 27:595-605, 1998.
16. Shah DM, Darling RC III, Chang BB, et al: Carotid endarterectomy by eversion technique: Its safety and durability. *Ann Surg* 228:471-478, 1998.
17. Bufo AJ, Shah DM, Chang BB, et al: Carotid bifurcationplasty: An alternative to patching. *J Cardiovasc Surg (Torino)* 33:308-310, 1992.

CHAPTER 5

Management of Carotid Kinks and Coils

Victor J. Weiss, M.D.
Fellow in Vascular Surgery, Division of Vascular Surgery, Emory
University School of Medicine, Atlanta, Georgia

Robert B. Smith III, M.D.
John E. Skandalakis Professor of Surgery, Division of Vascular Surgery,
Emory University School of Medicine, Atlanta, Georgia; Medical
Director, Emory University Hospital, Atlanta, Georgia

Reiser et al.[1] performed the first successful surgical correction of a tortuous extracranial carotid artery in 1951. Since that time, great progress has been made in the diagnosis and treatment of cerebrovascular disease. Despite these advances, the etiology of carotid tortuosity, the natural history of these findings, the indications for surgical correction, and the method of repair of the carotid kink or coil remain controversial.

The vascular surgeon is often confronted with a tortuous, coiled, or kinked carotid artery at the time of endarterectomy. In the days when contrast arteriography was the primary method of preoperative imaging, the surgeon would be aware of the tortuosity when entering the operation and could have a premeditated plan for carotid shortening. However, as imaging has shifted toward US as the lone modality, the surgeon is more likely to be surprised by the finding of a carotid kink or coil. For that reason, experienced vascular surgeons have a variety of techniques in their repertoire for repairing carotid kinks and redundancies. This article discusses several proven methods of carotid shortening and highlights those techniques we prefer.

INCIDENCE

Classification of carotid elongation was introduced by Weibel and Fields in 1965.[2] Based on their terminology, carotid tortuosity is defined as any *c*- or *s*-shaped elongation of the carotid artery, a coil is a circular configuration or exaggerated *s* shape, and a carotid kink is an abrupt angle in the artery associated with the potential for stenosis. The incidence of carotid elongation in patients undergoing cerebral arteriography is reported to be between 4% and 34% in adults[2-6] and between 15% and 43% in children.[2] The incidence of actual carotid kinking is 5% to 16%.[7]

ETIOLOGY

During maturation of the fetal neck, the carotid arteries straighten as the heart and great vessels descend into the mediastinum. The etiology of carotid elongation seen in children is related to maldescent of the heart during fetal development. This theory of congenital carotid coiling is supported by the finding that approximately 50% of cases of carotid redundancy in children are bilateral. Furthermore, other vascular anomalies such as aortic coarctation are associated with carotid coiling in children. Carotid coiling in the adult population is more commonly unilateral and is frequently associated with atherosclerotic degeneration. The resultant weakening of the arterial wall may predispose the vessel to elongation.

It is believed that carotid kinks are acquired, and that they are more likely to cause such neurologic symptoms as transient ischemic attacks, positional cerebral ischemia, or cerebral infarction. Such kinks are often associated with bifurcation atherosclerosis, elongation of the vessel, and even aneurysm formation. Most investigators agree that carotid kinks represent a greater risk for an ischemic stroke than either elongation or coiling of the internal carotid artery.

SIGNS AND SYMPTOMS

Isolated carotid coils (those not associated with atherosclerosis) have been implicated as an identifiable but infrequent source of cerebral ischemia, especially in children[8]; however, the carotid kink is the lesion that is more commonly responsible for neurologic manifestations. Related symptoms are thought to result from a temporary flow reduction related to excessive angulation at the site of bending. Flow reduction occurs most often when the head is turned sharply to one side, and axial torsion causes an accentuation of the kink. In most cases, ipsilateral rotation produces the greatest reduction in blood flow, but other head movements may have similar effects. A history of repetitive, focal neurologic deficits brought about by head movement should raise suspicion of carotid kinking. In addition, shear forces related to turbulent flow in the region of the kink may injure the endothelium, which would result in cerebrovascular embolization from platelet deposition.

A physical examination is often unrevealing in patients with carotid redundancy, but movement of the head may permit the carotid pulsation to become more pronounced. The earliest recognition of carotid kinks and coils as being clinically significant was as an alert from unsuspecting otolaryngologists who injured protruding vessels at the time of a tonsillectomy, adenoidectomy, or peritonsillar abscess incision.[9] Thus, palpation within the tonsillar fossa may allow detection of an excessively long, tortuous internal carotid artery. A carotid bruit may or may not be detectable.

DIAGNOSIS

The definitive test to diagnose carotid kinks and coils remains contrast angiography. Four-vessel cerebral angiography, including aortic arch and intracranial views, is necessary to exclude other associated vascular lesions. Imaging with the head in various positions of flexion, extension, and rotation may allow one to demonstrate an exacerbation of carotid elongation into a more pronounced kink or coil.

Currently, the most commonly used modality for the diagnosis of carotid occlusive disease is real-time B-mode Doppler US. The capability of this test to detect and quantify the degree of carotid stenosis has been well documented. B-mode US, however, is not an ideal test for detecting carotid tortuosity because distorted flow patterns and vessel angulation may produce Doppler frequency shifts that are difficult to interpret.

Oculoplethysmography (OPG) has been used as a noninvasive method for the detection of flow-limiting carotid kinks.[10] Although OPG may allow the confirmation of flow limitation with positional changes, the findings do not represent a reliable indication for or against surgery, as some with positive results continue to have symptoms after surgical correction and others with negative results have had alleviation of symptoms. Furthermore, this method has never been assessed in a blind, prospective fashion. Because of these shortcomings, OPG remains a rarely used test for the diagnosis of the hemodynamic significance of carotid kinking.

INDICATIONS FOR SURGERY

The generally accepted indications for the surgical correction of carotid kinks include evidence that the angulation may be responsible for neurologic symptoms as shown by the reproduction of focal neurologic findings with head movement, as well as the exclusion of other lesions that may produce similar symptoms.

Any patient with focal neurologic findings contralateral to a carotid kink should undergo surgical correction, even in the absence of demonstrable atheromatous disease if other causes for the neurologic findings are not found. This, however, is a rare occurrence.[4] Asymptomatic kinks, discovered as an incidental finding on arteriography, should be repaired if the kink produces a complete or nearly complete interruption of blood flow in the provocative position.

Carotid coils are similarly treated if suspected to be symptomatic and when all other causes of neurologic symptoms are excluded. The asymptomatic carotid coil should be followed with serial duplex examinations to detect areas of stenosis requiring endarterectomy, irrespective of the coil. Because the natural history of these relatively rare lesions is uncertain, one must remember that the benefit of surgical management for asymptomatic kinks and coils remains to be proven.

More commonly, patients undergoing carotid endarterectomies are discovered to have redundancy of the vessel with angulation at the apex of the rigid atheroma. After the endarterectomy, the atheromatous obstruction may be relieved, but one is left with a tortuous carotid artery that is capable of bending into a flow-limiting kink with resultant postoperative thrombosis. In addition, the vessel may be subjected to turbulent flow, platelet deposition, and subsequent accumulation of potentially embolic debris. For these reasons, we have adopted a liberal policy of shortening when an endarterectomy is performed in a setting of carotid elongation. In recent years, 10% to 15% of carotid operations performed by the senior author have had adjunctive shortening procedures.

SURGICAL MANAGEMENT

It is our preference to perform the vast majority of carotid operations using local anesthesia, including those operations on patients with carotid kinks and coils.[11] Additionally, nearly all patients undergo carotid shunting. One must use extreme care when passing the shunt into a tortuous carotid artery because intimal injury or arterial dissection may occur. If severe tortuosity exists high in the internal carotid artery, extra side holes may be cut into the shunt at the distal end, thereby ensuring flow in the event that the tip of the shunt abuts the vessel wall. All procedures aimed at straightening the redundant carotid artery require adequate mobilization of the adjacent common and internal carotid arteries. Dividing all tethering fibrous bands allows safe passage of the shunt, more accurate assessment of the carotid length, and a more precise shortening procedure. Because carotid kinks and coils are most often associated with atheromatous stenosis, an endarterectomy is very commonly needed. On occasion, atheromatous plaque may actually serve as a stent and, once removed, may result in carotid elongation. With the vessel fully mobilized and the shunt in place, the surgeon has several techniques of carotid shortening from which to choose. The method selected will depend on the segment of artery primarily affected and the preference of the individual surgeon.

The earliest documented procedure to straighten a redundant carotid artery involved suture fixation of the artery to the adjacent sternocleidomastoid muscle.[1] Even though this procedure was associated with a low stroke risk due to the vessel lumen not being entered, this technique is rarely, if ever, done today because modern treatment is directed at removing the associated atheromatous plaque and performing a concomitant shortening procedure by anastomosis or plication. Bypass of the tortuous segment with a vein graft or synthetic prosthesis has lost popularity because of a high rate of postoperative occlusion.

Resection of the elongated segment of the internal carotid artery with reanastomosis of the transected ends is a conceptually simple approach.[12] This technique, however, requires suture placement at the more distal internal carotid artery, which may be friable and may not hold sutures well. Resection of the redundant segment of the internal carotid artery and replacement with reversed saphenous vein has been preferred by some. This method avoids the potential of transforming a coil into a kink when using proximal reimplantation techniques. The major shortcoming involves creation of two anastomoses, including one in the more distal internal carotid artery that may be difficult to expose adequately.

An alternative technique involves resection of a cuff of the internal carotid artery and direct advancement for reattachment at the original location on the common carotid artery. Similarly, the elongated carotid artery may be transected at its origin, then anastomosed to a location more proximal on the common carotid artery. Although technically sound, these methods often require the addition of a patch to ensure an adequate luminal diameter.

Our preferred method of shortening the internal carotid artery typically involves endarterectomy, followed by proximal transection of the redundant vessel. The internal carotid artery is divided obliquely, which leaves the posterior wall longer than the anterior wall. The vessel is then rotated 180 degrees, which allows the posterior wall of the internal carotid artery to act as a patch extending onto the anterior aspect of the common carotid artery (Fig 1). Frequently, the internal carotid patch is shorter than the length of the arteriotomy. In this instance, the more proximal segment of common carotid artery may be closed primarily. This technique,

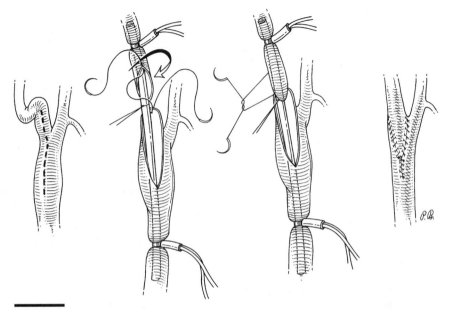

FIGURE 1.
Shortening of the internal carotid artery. After endarterectomy, the internal carotid artery is transected in an oblique fashion. Anastomosis is performed with 180-degree rotation of the internal carotid artery, which functions as a patch angioplasty. The proximal portion of the common carotid artery may be approximated primarily.

similar to others described by Chino[13] and Hamann,[14] allows precise shortening and simultaneous creation of an autogenous patch.

When appropriate, shortening of the common carotid artery may be easier because this vessel has a thicker wall and holds sutures more readily. It is feasible when both the internal and external branches are buckled and, therefore, eligible to be straightened. The common carotid artery may be treated by resection of a segment of common carotid artery and end-to-end anastomosis. The method espoused by Quattelbaum et al.[15] involved resection of the carotid bifurcation and ligation of the external carotid artery. Most surgeons currently prefer those alternative approaches that spare the external carotid artery and the potential collateral vessels arising from it. Our preference is to maintain the bifurcation and the external carotid artery intact and to plicate the adjacent common carotid artery by imbricating the posterior and lateral walls with a continuous monofilament suture. The carotid arteriotomy may then be patched or primarily closed at the discretion of the surgeon (Fig 2).

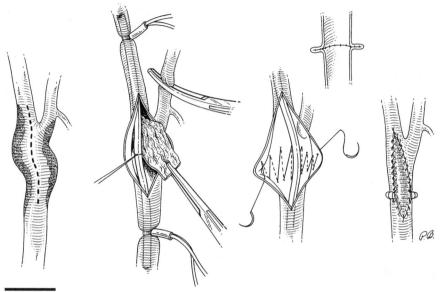

FIGURE 2.
Plication of the redundant common carotid artery. After endarterectomy, the lateral and posterior walls are plicated with a continuous, monofilament suture. A patch may be added at the discretion of the surgeon.

CONCLUSION

The symptomatic kink or coil has become a well-accepted albeit infrequent indication for carotid artery shortening. The natural history of the asymptomatic kink, or the carotid artery left redundant, after endarterectomy is poorly understood. Conceptually, any tortuous vessel that exhibits postoperative turbulence could ultimately thicken as a result of altered flow dynamics. If associated with a turbulent or reduced flow as a consequence of being elongated or kinked, the artery that has recently undergone endarterectomy is at least theoretically vulnerable to platelet deposition. Therefore, it makes intuitive sense that these vessels should be left with straight-line, fully patent flow. Because these beliefs are not borne out by scientific study, it is imperative that any method of carotid shortening be free of additional morbidity when combined with carotid endarterectomy. It has, in fact, been demonstrated that adding a variety of shortening procedures to an endarterectomy does not increase morbidity or mortality when compared with an endarterectomy without shortening.[11,13,15-17] Additionally, carotid shortening has not been found to increase late morbidity (i.e., a higher restenosis rate) when compared with endarterectomy alone.[11]

In summary, isolated elongation of the carotid artery, either as a kink or coil, may occasionally be responsible for producing neurologic symptoms. More commonly, one is confronted with arterial redundancy at the time of a carotid endarterectomy. Vascular surgeons should have in their armamentarium several techniques to shorten the carotid artery, thereby producing both a safe and hemodynamically favorable reconstruction.

REFERENCES

1. Reiser MM, Geraud J, Ducoudray J, et al: Dolicho-internal carotid with vertiginous syndrome. *Rev Neurol* 85:145-147, 1951.
2. Weibel J, Fields WS: Tortuosity, coiling, and kinking of the internal carotid artery: I. Etiology and radiographic anatomy. *Neurology* 15:7-11, 1965.
3. Cioffi FA, Meduri M, Tomasello F, et al: Kinking and coiling of the internal carotid artery: Clinical–statistical observations and surgical perspectives. *J Neurol Surg Sci* 19:15-22, 1975.
4. Perdue GD, Barreca JP, Smith RB: The significance of elongation and angulation of the carotid artery: A negative view. *Surgery* 77:45-52, 1975.
5. Metz H, Murray-Leslie RM, Bannister RG: Kinking of the internal carotid artery in relation to cerebrovascular disease. *Lancet* 1:424-426, 1961.
6. Bauer R, Sheehan S, Meyer JS: Arteriographic study of cerebrovascular disease: II. Cerebral symptoms due to kinking, tortuosity and compression of carotid and vertebral arteries in the neck. *Arch Neurol* 4:119-131, 1961.
7. Vannix RS, Joergenson FJ, Carter R: Kinking of the internal carotid artery. Clinical significance and surgical management. *Am J Surg* 134:82-89, 1977.
8. Sakari NBS, Holmes JM, Bickerstaff ER: Neurologic manifestations associated with carotid loops and kinks in children. *J Neurol Neurosurg Psychiatry* 33:194-200, 1970.
9. Fisher AGT: Sigmoid tortuosity of the internal carotid artery and its relation to tonsil and pharynx. *Lancet* 2:128-130, 1915.
10. Stanton PE, McClusky DA, Lamis PA: Hemodynamic assessment and surgical correction of kinking of the internal carotid artery. *Surgery* 84:793-797, 1978.
11. Coyle KA, Smith RB III, Chapman RL, et al: Carotid artery shortening: A safe adjunct to carotid endarterectomy. *J Vasc Surg* 22:257-263, 1995.
12. Hsu I, Kisten AD: Buckling of the great vessels. *Arch Intern Med* 98:712-714, 1956.
13. Chino ES: A simple method for combined carotid endarterectomy and correction of internal carotid artery kinking. *J Vasc Surg* 6:197-199, 1987.
14. Hamann H: Carotid endarterectomy: Prevention of stroke in asymptomatic (stage I) and symptomatic (stage II) patients. *Thorac Cardiovasc Surg* 36:272-275, 1988.

15. Quattelbaum JK Jr, Upson ET, Neville RL: Strokes associated with elongation and kinking of the internal carotid artery. *Ann Surg* 150:824-832, 1959.

16. Collins PS, Orecchia P, Gomez E: A technique for correction of carotid kinks and coils following endarterectomy. *Ann Vasc Surg* 5:116-120, 1991.

17. Archie JP: Carotid endarterectomy with reconstruction techniques tailored to operative findings. *J Vasc Surg* 17:141-151, 1993.

PART II
Aortic Disease

CHAPTER 6

Endovascular Treatment of Abdominal Aortic Aneurysms

Gregorio A. Sicard, M.D.
Professor of Surgery, Washington University School of Medicine, Chief, Division of General Surgery and Section of Vascular Surgery, Barnes-Jewish Hospital, St. Louis, Missouri

Brian G. Rubin, M.D.
Assistant Professor of Surgery, Washington University School of Medicine, Barnes-Jewish Hospital, St. Louis, Missouri

Rupture of an abdominal aortic aneurysm (AAA) is the cause of death for more than 15,000 Americans each year. The overall mortality of aneurysm rupture exceeds 90% when prehospital and inpatient mortality is combined. Currently, there is no effective medical therapy to reduce the rate of aneurysm growth or rupture. Until recently, the only effective treatment of AAAs was measurement and monitoring of aneurysm size with elective open surgical repair. More than 45,000 patients undergo elective infrarenal aortic aneurysm repair each year in an effort to prevent AAA rupture, making this the second most commonly performed vascular surgical operation. Although most centers report excellent outcomes after open AAA repair, the procedure is associated with significant postoperative discomfort and morbidity, as well as a prolonged recovery period. Driven by the combination of patient, physician, and medical industry interests, an endovascular approach to AAA repair has resulted in an explosive development and investigation of multiple devices. Although the majority of practicing vascular surgeons has yet to implant one of these grafts, the concepts of device design, results of clinical trials, and complications of endovascular AAA repair are of keen interest to the vascular surgery community. In the near future, several of the endovascular devices developed and tested for AAA repair will be released for general use by appropriately trained physicians.

HISTORICAL PERSPECTIVE

Investigation into the feasibility of endoluminal graft placement began in 1976 by Juan Parodi. Initially unsuccessful, Parodi's interest in endovascular AAA repair was rekindled in the 1980s after development of the endoluminal stent by Julio Palmaz. The concept of a graft anchored to the aortic wall by an endoluminal stent was conceived, and the first "homemade" stent-grafts were constructed. The era of human endovascular AAA repair was ushered in on September 6, 1990, when a 70-year-old patient with severe chronic obstructive pulmonary disease and a 6-cm AAA underwent successful implantation via a femoral arteriotomy of a balloon-expandable stent attached to a tubular knitted Dacron graft. The initial report by Parodi et al.[1] included five patients treated for AAA, aortic dissection, or spontaneous atheroembolism. At first, their stent-graft had only a single cephalad stent, but by the third patient, persistent blood flow around the distal end of the graft was noted. The fourth patient received a distal stent to exclude flow into the aneurysm sac. Parodi's insightful report of endovascular AAA repair noted several limitations and concerns, all of which remain salient today. These included (1) stent-graft migration, (2) endoleaks both at attachment sites and from patent lumbar and inferior mesenteric arteries, (3) embolization of aortic thrombus, (4) the anatomical constraints of an AAA, allowing placement of tube grafts only, and (5) the importance of iliac diameter and tortuosity in allowing transfemoral access to the abdominal aorta.

Despite initial promise in concept, less than 10% of AAA patients had aortic anatomy suitable to placement of an endovascular tube graft, usually because of an insufficient segment of distal aorta onto which the graft could be anchored. In 1995, Chuter et al.[2] described their initial results of endovascular AAA exclusion in 22 patients treated with a bifurcated prosthesis. A cross-femoral catheter was used to pull one graft limb over the aortic bifurcation and into position in the iliac artery contralateral from the side of device introduction. Despite a steep learning curve associated with early complications, most patients underwent successful placement of the bifurcated device. The sole mortality in their series was from aneurysm rupture caused by a distal graft attachment site leak that resulted in arterial pressurization of the AAA.

Aorto-uni-iliac endovascular grafting was described in Parodi's initial report in 1991.[1] In 1995, Chuter in association with surgeons of University Hospital Nottingham in England emphasized the indications and technique of aorto-uni-iliac graft placement with femorofemoral bypass.[3] Patients without a suitable distal aortic neck for tube graft placement, or with a single wide or aneurysmal iliac artery were considered candidates for this approach. Yusuf et al.[3] deployed an aorto-uni-iliac stent-graft, embolized and occluded the contralateral common iliac artery, and restored contralateral limb perfusion with a femorofemoral bypass. Their report emphasized the rapid recovery associated with endoluminal AAA repair, with their first patient having resumed a standard diet within 24 hours after surgery.

These initial reports of success prompted both corporations and medical centers to focus intense efforts on the design, fabrication, and implantation of endoluminal devices in the aorta. As a consequence, several homemade and manufactured endovascular AAA devices are currently being implanted as part of clinical trials. On February 10, 1993, the initial North American implantation of a manufactured endoluminal graft began with a device produced by Endovascular Technologies, Inc (Menlo Park, Calif) based on a design by Harrison M. Lazarus. This initial work was a Food and Drug Administration (FDA)–approved phase I trial to demonstrate device safety and technical feasibility in good-risk AAA patients. Three years later, Moore and Rutherford[4] described 46 patients treated with implantation, in whom the success rate was 85%, the average operating time was 194 minutes, limited perioperative complications occurred, and no patients died.

CHARACTERISTICS OF ENDOVASCULAR AAA GRAFTS

One of the most competitive areas in biomedical engineering has been the development of the optimal endovascular graft for AAA repair. The devices differ in their attachment systems, graft material and support, modularity, and size of access required.[5,6] The principal features of the grafts currently undergoing investigation in the United States are summarized in Table 1.

ATTACHMENT SYSTEMS

The devices in clinical trials base their attachment systems on a self-expanding metal stent system. Conceptually, grafts based on self-expanding systems might be able to radially dilate with continued expansion of the aorta at the attachment sites. Once the initial stent–attachment system deployment has occurred, the stents are ballooned firmly against the aortic wall. The AnCure graft (Guidant/Endovascular Technologies [EVT]) has a metal frame

TABLE 1.

Features of Endoluminal Grafts Currently Under Investigation in the United States

Name	Company	Profile French (mm)	Device Type	Attachment System	Graft Features	FDA Study Phase
AnCure	Guidant/EVT	27 (9.0)	Single unit	Self-expanding with hooks	Unsupported Dacron graft	III
Vanguard	Boston Scientific	22 (7.3)	Modular	Self-expanding nitinol	Nitinol frame on luminal surface	II
AneuR$_x$	Medtronic	22 (7.3)	Modular	Self-expanding nitinol	Nitinol exoskeleton	III
Corvita	Boston Scientific	18 (6.0)	Modular	Self-expanding braided wire	Self-expanding braided wire exoskeleton, "spun" polyurethane graft, both legs modular	I→II
Excluder	W.L. Gore	18 (6.0)	Modular	Self-expanding nitinol	ePTFE with nitinol frame	II
Talent	World Medical	22-24 (7.8)	Modular	Self-expanding nitinol	Dacron graft, nitinol skeleton inside body and outside limbs	III
Zenith	Cook	19 (6.3)	Modular	Gianturco Z-stent, top stent with barbs	Dacron	Phase I sites chosen
Baxter	Baxter	18 (6.0)	Modular	Self-expanding Elgilay	Dacron	II

Abbreviations: FDA, Food and Drug Administration; *EVT*, Endovascular Technologies; *ePTFE*, expanded thin polytetrafluoroethylene.

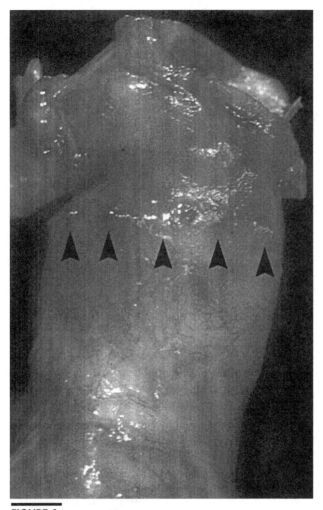

FIGURE 1.
The proximal attachment system of the EVT AnCure device has hooks that penetrate deeply into the aortic wall. The hooks can be seen from the external surface of the aorta (*arrowheads*). Also note the proximity of the stent to the renal arteries in this autopsy specimen.

with attachment hooks that penetrate into the aortic wall, providing firm fixation to prevent distal migration (Fig 1). Other graft-attachment designs rely on similar hooks, barbs, or the graft exoskeleton to resist longitudinal compression or displacement by blood flow. Most devices require a proximal aortic neck of approximately 1.5 cm in length. Some endografts such as the Talent graft (World Medical Manufacturing Corp, Sunrise, Fla) has an uncovered proximal stent with wide interstices to permit the proximal attachment site to be placed in the suprarenal position if necessary. In contrast to these self-expanding stent-graft designs, balloon-expandable stents, as attachment anchors are more difficult to deploy initially, but are used in most homemade stent-graft designs.

GRAFT SUPPORT SYSTEMS

Aneurysm formation involves elongation of the aortoiliac segment as well as radial expansion. As a consequence of this elongation, significant tortuosity may be present on both the aorta and iliac systems. Vessel tortuosity can result in kinking of endografts that are not supported along their length. Most of the endografts currently under investigation contain a graft "skeleton" to reduce kinks or wrinkles along the length of the graft. After graft placement, completion aortography, intravascular US, or both may be used to ensure that the graft contains no significantly enfolding that would impair blood flow or predispose to graft limb thrombosis. In addition, the device exoskeleton serves to supply additional column strength to increase graft resistance to longitudinal shortening.

GRAFT MATERIAL

All devices in the American trials are made of one of three materials: Dacron (polyester) typically woven ultrathin to 0.1- to 0.3-mm thickness, expanded thin polytetrafluoroethylene (ePTFE), or polycarbonate (spun polyurethane). Manufacturers have selected these materials because of their proven clinical acceptability as aortic grafts or because they allow design of low-profile devices. For some of the newer graft designs, a thin layer of graft material is applied over or bonded to the graft skeleton, minimizing implant diameter while maintaining nonporous characteristics.

MODULAR VERSUS SINGLE-UNIT DESIGN

Graft design can be characterized by whether a single component comprises the entire graft, or whether the final endograft is composed of pieces (modular design) that are overlapped and assembled inside the aorta (Fig 2). Only the AnCure graft is based on a single-unit design. Single-unit grafts require careful preoperative imaging studies to manufacture a graft of predetermined length between the proximal and distal attachment sites. In contrast, modular graft designs allow some flexibility in the overall graft length, either by changing the overlap distance of the components, or by adding extenders at the proximal or distal attachment sites or "landing zones" of the graft. This adaptability allows modular grafts to be constructed by assembly of graft

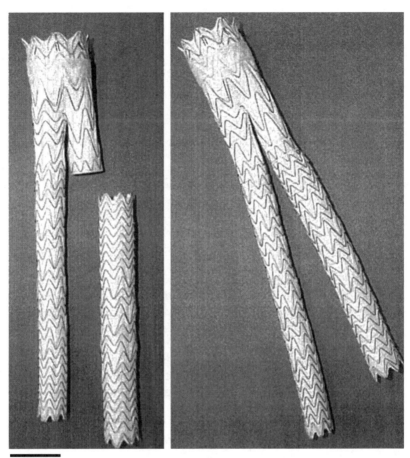

FIGURE 2.
Modular endovascular grafts come as separate units that are assembled inside the aorta. The separate pieces of the Gore Excluder graft are shown apart **(left)** and assembled **(right)**. Also note the external skeleton of this graft, which provides support against longitudinal and radial compressive forces.

pieces of standard sizes, without the need to manufacture a graft for each specific patient.

DELIVERY SYSTEMS

Introducing the stent-graft in its delivery system via a femoral arteriotomy can prove challenging. Stenosis and tortuosity of the iliac arteries are the principal problems confronting the surgeon. The primary introducer mechanism is placed through the less diseased and tortuous iliac vessel. Predilation of focal stenoses is occasionally required to obtain endovascular access to the aorta. For the large introducer sheath required for the AnCure device (27F), we have used a series of Amplatz renal dilators (Amplatz Urological, Spencer, Indianapolis) to predilate the entire length of the ipsilateral iliac artery to a size adequate to allow device introduction. Iliac artery tortuosity is a problem, made worse if the introducer system or device is not flexible. Placement of a stiff guide wire will occasionally straighten the iliac vessels sufficiently to allow endograft placement. We have also carried out extensive dissection of the external iliac artery from the groin incision, and using longitudinal traction, the iliac system can be straightened enough to allow advancement of the introducer mechanism. Because problems with the iliac arterial segment are common, graft manufacturers have emphasized device designs with a low profile (i.e., a small diameter). Low-profile devices also have the potential to allow percutaneous graft placement rather than requiring an open, "surgical" arteriotomy.

DEPLOYMENT SYSTEMS

After successful passage of the device and its positioning within the aorta, the endograft is deployed. Typically this involves drawing back the sheath used for device introduction, releasing the constrained endograft, and allowing the attachment system to impact the aortic wall. Subsequent balloon inflation within the device lumen is used to anchor the graft attachment zones firmly to the artery wall. The mechanisms that result in graft deployment are designed to minimize operator error, prevent graft movement, and allow precise deployment. Examples of these types of mechanisms include the Gore Excluder "rip-cord" deployment system (W.L. Gore, Flagstaff, Ariz) or the Medtronic AneuR$_x$ "fishing reel" release system (Medtronic, Inc, Minneapolis, Minn).

SELECTION OF PATIENTS FOR ENDOVASCULAR AAA REPAIR

In healthy patients, open AAA repair can be performed with a perioperative mortality of 3% to 5%.[7] However, the postoperative period is marked by significant patient discomfort, a prolonged (5-7 day) hospital stay, and limitations in physical and social activity for several months. For good-risk surgical patients, the primary advantages of endovascular AAA repair are an expedited recovery with significantly reduced postoperative pain. Most of the devices are being evaluated in good-risk surgical patients, with a control arm in each trial consisting of patients undergoing open surgical repair. For poor-risk patients, open surgical repair is associated with mortality rates of up to 60%. For these patients, an endovascular approach performed under local or regional anesthesia presumably offers lower perioperative risk. Although no randomized trials have yet documented improvements in outcomes for high-risk patients, almost certainly this patient group will benefit the most from endovascular AAA repair, allowing otherwise untreatable patients to be considered as surgical candidates. Currently, the Talent graft in the United States is the only device with an FDA investigation device exemption allowing use in high-risk AAA patients.

Certain anatomical constraints limit application of an endovascular approach to all patients with AAA. For each device, specific criteria have been identified that must be fulfilled before patient enrollment in the device trial. General criteria include an adequate length of normal artery to allow proximal and distal graft attachment, typically 1.5 cm of infrarenal aortic neck. The attachment sites must be free of thrombus so the graft can be firmly impacted into the aortic and iliac vessel wall. As described above, the iliac vessels must be of acceptable caliber and without excessive tortuosity to allow endograft passage into the aortic segment. Some AAA endografts also place limits on the extent of aortic angulation within the infrarenal aorta, or between the suprarenal aorta and aneurysm neck. Finally, no vital vessels can originate in the portion of the aortoiliac system covered by the graft. An important accessory renal artery, inferior mesenteric artery, or both iliac arteries that would be covered after endograft placement contraindicates endoluminal AAA repair. In certain anatomical situations, preoperative or intraoperative endoluminal unilateral coil embolization of an internal iliac artery may be required to extend one limb of the endoluminal graft to the ipsilateral external iliac artery (Fig 3).

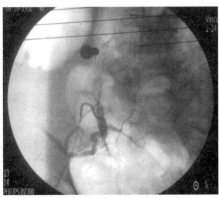 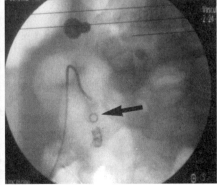

FIGURE 3.
Cannulation of right internal iliac artery (**left**) and coil embolization (**right,** *arrow*) in a patient with abdominal aortic and right common iliac artery aneurysms. Postcoil embolization, patient underwent an aorto–right external iliac, left common iliac EVT bifurcation endoluminal graft. *Abbreviation: EVT,* Endovascular Technologies.

RESULTS OF ENDOVASCULAR AAA REPAIR
TECHNICAL SUCCESS AND MORTALITY

A critical evaluation of endoluminal stent-covered grafts for the treatment of infrarenal AAA has been hampered by multiple factors: (1) continuous modification of devices (moving-target technology), (2) publications of series in which the results of multiple devices are combined, and (3) the lack of long-term results. Reports from investigators in Europe, Australia, and the United States have documented excellent technical success rates, a low incidence of conversion to open surgical repair, and a procedure mortality comparable to conventional surgical repair (Table 2).[8-12] Blum et al.[9] reported a large single-center experience with the Stentor-Vanguard device with excellent technical and short-term results. In the United States, recent experience with the phase II data of multicenter trials with the EVT/Guidant and AneuR$_x$/ Medtronic devices have been published.[13,14] The technical success rate with these two devices was equally excellent, with a postoperative mortality comparable to or lower than standard historical open-repair results in European and American series. In the EVT-Guidant as well as the Medtronic (AneuR$_x$) multicenter trials, the endoluminal graft postoperative mortality was also comparable to that of the open-repair control group in each series, respectively. Phase I data from the Gore/Excluder device also showed promising early results, which has led to the approval by the FDA for a phase II trial. Other devices, such as the Corvita-Schneider device and the Talent (Boston Scientific Medical Corp, Sunnise, Florida) device, have recently completed phase I and phase II trial data evaluation with similarly good early technical success and low mortality rates. Most investigators are in agreement that this technology will have a significant role in the treatment of AAAs. Until long-term results and improved versions of the current devices are available for evaluation, the exact impact of this technology remains a source of speculation, with predictions of 30% to 70% of infrarenal aneurysms treated in this manner in the next 5 years. In 1998 at our institution, 34% of all infrarenal aortic aneurysms were treated endoluminally.[15] We expect that approximately 50% will be treated endoluminally in the current year.

COMPLICATIONS

Endoleaks remain the Achilles' heel of AAAs (Table 3). White et al.[16] have recommended a classification for endoleaks in an attempt to stratify the source of the leak and hopefully, evaluate the natural history and long-term effects of early and late endoleaks (Table 4). Despite this classification, a number of endoleaks defy localization, making their significance a predica-

TABLE 2.
Results of Endovascular Stent-Graft Repair of AAAs: Selected Series

Author (Year)	No. of Patients	Type of Study	Devices Used	Technical Success	Open Conversion	Mortality (30-Day)
Stelter et al.[8] (1997)	201	Single center	Stentor-Vanguard Talent	178 (89%)	4 (2%)	7 (3.5%)
Blum et al.[9] (1997)	154	Single center	Stentor-Mintec	134 (87%)	3 (1.9%)	1 (0.6%)
May et al.[10] (1998)	108	Single center	Modified Parodi-EVT, White Yu, Mintec Stentor Chuter	95 (88%)	13 (12%)	3 (3%)
Coppi et al.[11] (1998)	66	Multicenter	Stentor-Mintec	60 (91%)	4 (6.1%)	1 (1.5%)
Harris et al.[12] (1998)	430	Multicenter-EUROSTAR	Stentor-Vanguard	420 (98%)	10 (2.3%)	14 (3.2%)
Goldstone et al.[13] (1998)	200	Multicenter	EVT	183 (92%)	17 (8.5%)	2 (1%)
Zarins et al.[14] (1999)	190	Multicenter	Medtronic-AneuR$_x$	185 (97%)	0 (0%)	5 (2.6%)
Authors' experience[15] (1999)	64	Single center	EVT	62 (97%)	2 (3%)	1 (1.6%)

Abbreviation: AAAs, abdominal aortic aneurysms; EVT, Endovascular Technologies.

TABLE 3.
Results of Endovascular Stent-Graft Repair of AAAs: Endoleaks

Author (Year)	No. of Patients	Follow-up CT	Early			Late			
			Attachment Site	Branch Flow	Indeterminate	Follow-up CT (mo)	Attachment Site	Branch Flow	Indeterminate
Stelter et al.[8] (1997)	201	3 months	18 (9%)	—	—	3-12	14 (7%)	3 (1.5%)	2 (1%)
Blum et al.[9] (1997)	154	Discharge	17 (11%)	—	—	—	4 (2.6%)	3 (2%)	—
May et al.[10] (1998)	108	Within 10 days	7 (6.5%)	—	—	6-36	6 (5.5%)	—	—
Coppi et al.[11] (1998)	66	3 months	4 (6%)	—	—	5-20	6 (9%)	—	—
Harris et al.[12] (1998)	430	—	68 (15.7%)	—	—	—	27 (6.3%)	—	—
EVT-Guidant* (1999)	174	Discharge	7 (4%)	62 (35.6%)	9 (5.2%)	12	0 (0%)	21 (30.9%)	2 (2.9%)
Zarins et al.[14] (1999)	185	Discharge	17 (9.2%)	2 (6.5%)	10 (5.4%)	12	—	2/33 (6%)	—
Authors' experience[15] (1999)	64	Discharge	6 (9.4%)	9 (14%)	—	6	1/50 (2%)	2/50 (4%)	—

*Guidant EndoVascular Technologies: Clinical study of the AnCure Tube and Bifurcated Systems extended indications evaluation. Unpublished data.

Abbreviation: AAAs, abdominal aortic aneurysms; *EVT,* Endovascular Technologies.

TABLE 4.
Classification of Endoleaks

Type I	Graft-related endoleak (attachment site or "transgraft")
	IA: Perigraft or transgraft endoleak with no identified outflow
	IB: Perigraft or transgraft endoleak with lumbar or inferior mesenteric outflow.
Type II	Retrograde or branch flow endoleak
	IA: Retrograde endoleak with no outflow
	IB: Retrograde endoleak with outflow channels

(Modified from White GH, May J, Waugh RC, et al: Type I and type II endoleaks: A more useful classification for reported results of endoluminal AAA repair. *J Endovasc Surg* 5:189-193, 1998.)

ment. In the European multicenter study of endovascular repair of AAA, predischarge endoleaks were detected by CT scan in 66 (15.7%) of 430 patients.[17] Late development of endoleaks was identified in an additional 27 patients (6.3%). Of importance was the finding of an increase in the maximum transverse diameter of the excluded aneurysm in 11.4% of patients with no endoleaks compared with 53.3% of those with endoleaks. In our experience with 64 patients (66 devices) and a mean follow-up of 12 months, we have not observed any patient with growth of their aneurysm. Some patients have had spectacular regression or disappearance of the aneurysm (Fig 4). Other investigators have noted high endoleak rates if the postoperative CT scan is obtained in the immediate postoperative period compared with a 30-day CT scan. Leaks across the graft material as well as many branch flow leaks will seal spontaneously in the first 30 days. Late-appearing endoleaks may represent absorption of the thrombus and appearance of delayed branch flow. Occasionally, the lumbar arteries or the inferior mesenteric artery can serve as early or late outflow to a periprosthetic leak (Fig 5).

Many approaches have been suggested to attempt to resolve attachment site as well as branch flow endoleaks. Most investigators agree that if a significant attachment site leak is identified at operation, every possible maneuver should be exhausted to seal the endoleak. This may include the introduction of a second device in the single-unit EVT or the use of extenders in the modular devices. In our experience with 64 patients, 6 (9.4%) have had attachment site leaks. Two proximal aortic attachment leaks were resolved successfully intraoperatively by implantation of a second device. Three small iliac attachment site leaks resolved sponta-

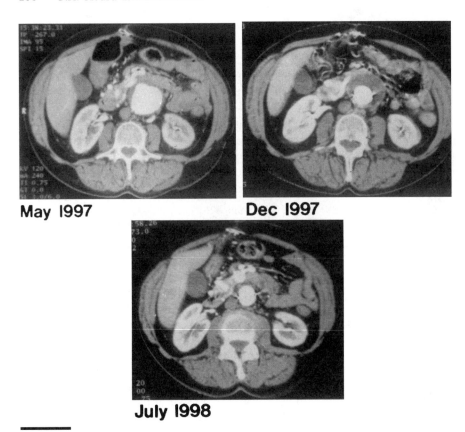

May 1997   Dec 1997

July 1998

FIGURE 4.
CT follow-up in patient who underwent endoluminal (EVT) repair of 5.4-cm aneurysm in May 1997. Note disappearance of the aneurysm sac by July 1998. *Abbreviation: EVT,* Endovascular Technologies.

neously and one required open surgical repair of the iliac limb. Should intraluminal perioperative maneuvers fail to seal large attachment leaks, strong consideration should be given to open conversion. Residual small attachment leaks must be followed up closely with a repeated CT scan within 3 months. If the periprosthetic endoleak is identified on the postoperative CT scan and duplex US, attempts to seal by endoluminal techniques have been successful, although occasionally require open conversion if the device used has no extenders. For lumbar or inferior mesenteric artery retrograde endoleaks, various approaches have been suggested including a "watchful waiting" as the endoleak resolves in most cases, postoperative endoluminal coil embolization, insertion of thrombogenic substances in the aneurysmal sac, and laparoscopic clipping of the inferior mesenteric artery or lumbar artery. Most early reports suggest that the great majority of branch

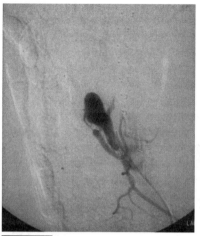 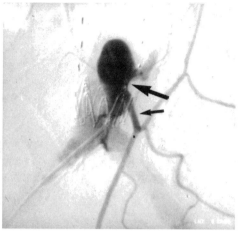

FIGURE 5.
Distal attachment site endoleak detected in follow-up CT scan **(left).** Arteriogram **(right)** demonstrates the distal attachment site leak (*large arrow*) and outflow through patent inferior mesenteric artery (*small arrow*).

flow endoleaks will seal spontaneously. If there is persistent branch flow for more than 3 months, options to consider are coil embolization of the lumbar arteries in continuity with the hypogastric circulation. In cases of a distal attachment site leak, embolization of the branch leak through the attachment site followed by embolization, and balloon angioplasty of the attachment site can resolve the leak. Laparoscopic clipping of the persistent lumbar or inferior mesenteric artery type II endoleaks and laparoscopic banding of type I endoleaks have been anecdotally reported, with no significant series available to evaluate their merit.

Another device-related complication is limb dysfunction usually caused by kinking or external compression. This complication is more frequent in the EVT/Guidant device because of the lack of external limb support. Any kinking or external compression of a limb detected in the completion arteriogram can be easily resolved by endoluminal placement of a WallStent (Fig 6). Occasionally limb dysfunction is detected in the postoperative period by a decrease in the ankle-brachial index. Arteriographic confirmation of the stenotic area can lead to endoluminal treatment and restoration of normal graft limb patency (Fig 7).

Longitudinal shrinkage of the aneurysm has been the source of late complications in some of the modular devices.[18] This physical change in the aorta and iliac arteries can lead to migration from the proximal or distal attachment sites from the native arteries, separation of modular components, kinking of limbs

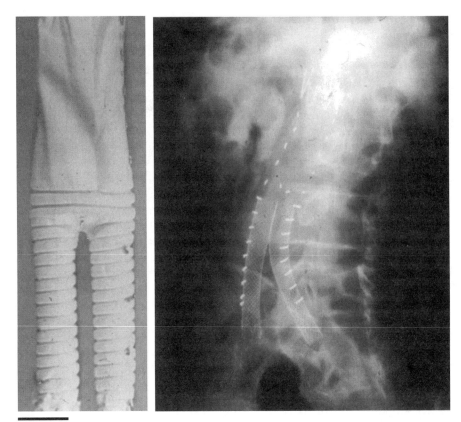

FIGURE 6.
Bifurcated EVT endoluminal stent-graft showing no support in the limbs **(left).**
Bilateral Wall Stents in bifurcated EVT graft **(right)** for compression of both limbs,
creating a gradient across the iliac limbs. *Abbreviation: EVT,* Endovascular
Technologies.

with subsequent thrombosis, and rarely fracture of the stent
with perforation of the fabric and an acute "transgraft" leak.
These complications primarily have been reported in the modular device experience. New generations of modular devices
should be designed to not only resist the constant mechanical
stresses, but also to respond to longitudinal shrinkage of the
aorta.

SUMMARY

The endoluminal repair of infrarenal aortic aneurysms is a promising procedure that is still in evolution. The excellent short-term
results are very encouraging. The lack of long-term results, as well
as the incidence of late-appearing complications, indicate that this
technology should still be considered investigational. The critical
evaluation by controlled clinical trials of the current devices will

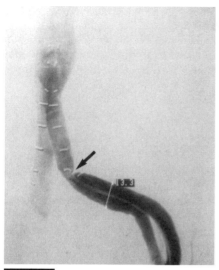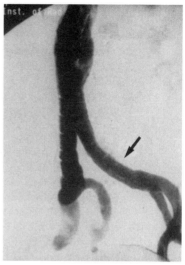

FIGURE 7.
Delayed stenosis of left iliac limb of bifurcated endoluminal graft detected by abnormal ankle/arm indices **(left)**. Patient treated endoluminally successfully with a WallStent **(right)**.

lead to the identification of problems that must be resolved if this technology is to have a significant impact in the treatment of AAAs.

REFERENCES

1. Parodi JCL, Palmaz JCL, Barone HD: Transfemoral intraluminal graft implantation for abdominal aortic aneurysms. *Ann Vasc Surg* 5:491-499, 1991.
2. Chuter TA, Wendt G, Hopkinson BR, et al: Transfemoral insertion of a bifurcated endovascular graft for aortic aneurysm repair: The first 22 patients. *Cardiovasc Surg* 3:121-128, 1995.
3. Yusuf SW, Baker DM, Hind RE, et al: Endoluminal transfemoral abdominal aortic aneurysm repair with aorto-uni-iliac graft and femorofemoral bypass. *Br J Surg* 82:916, 1995.
4. Moore WS, Rutherford RB: Transfemoral endovascular repair of abdominal aortic aneurysm: Results of the North American EVT phase 1 trial. *J Vasc Surg* 23:543-553, 1996.
5. Ohki T, Veith FJ, Sanchez LA, et al: Varying strategies and devices for endovascular repair of abdominal aortic aneurysms. *Semin Vasc Surg* 10:242-256, 1997.
6. Marin M, Hollier LH: Endovascular grafts. *Semin Vasc Surg* 12:64-73, 1999.
7. Ernst CB: Abdominal aortic aneurysms. *N Engl J Med* 328:1167-1172, 1993.
8. Stelter W, Umscheid T, Ziegler P: Three-year experience with modular stent-graft devices for endovascular AAA treatment. *J Endovasc Surg* 4:362-369, 1997.

9. Blum U, Voshage G, Lammer J, et al: Endoluminal stent-grafts for infrarenal abdominal aortic aneurysms. *N Engl J Med* 336:13-20, 1997.

10. May J, White GH, Yu W, Cameron NL, et al: Concurrent comparison of endoluminal versus open repair in the treatment of abdominal aortic aneurysms: Analysis of 303 patients by life table method. *J Vasc Surg* 27:213-221, 1998.

11. Coppi G, Pacchioni R, Moratto R, et al: Experience with the Stentor endograft at four Italian centers. *J Endovasc Surg* 5:206-215, 1998.

12. Harris PL, Gilling-Smith GL, Buth J: Latest figures from the EUROSTAR registry. *J Endovasc Surg* 5:172A, 1998.

13. Goldstone J, Brewster DC, Chaikof EL, et al: Endoluminal repair versus standard open repair of abdominal aortic aneurysms: Early results of a prospective clinical comparison trial. Presented at the 46th Scientific Meeting of the North American Chapter of the International Society for Cardiovascular Surgery, San Diego, June 1998.

14. Zarins CK, White RA, Schwarten D, et al: AneuRx stent graft versus open surgical repair of abdominal aortic aneurysms: Multicenter prospective clinical trial. *J Vasc Surg* 29:292-308, 1999.

15. Sicard GA, Allen BT, Rubin BG, et al: Unpublished data.

16. White GH, May J, Waugh RC, et al: Type I and type II endoleaks: A more useful classification for reported results of endoluminal AAA repair. *J Endovasc Surg* 5:189-193, 1998.

17. Gilling-Smith GL, Cuypers P, Buth J, et al: The significance of endoleaks after endovascular AAA repair: Results of a large European multicenter study. *J Endovasc Surg* 5:I-1A-I-40A, 1998.

18. Harris P, Brennan J, Martin J, et al: Longitudinal aneurysm shrinkage following endovascular aortic aneurysm repair: A source of intermediate and late complications. *J Endovasc Surg* 6:11-16, 1999.

CHAPTER 7

How and When to Treat an Endoleak After Endovascular Abdominal Aortic Aneurysm Repair

Bert C. Eikelboom, M.D.
Associate Professor of Vascular Surgery, University of Utrecht; Chief, Department of Vascular Surgery, University Hospital Utrecht, Utrecht, The Netherlands

Jan D. Blankensteijn, M.D.
Professor of Vascular Surgery, University of Utrecht; Consultant Vascular Surgeon, Department of Vascular Surgery, University Hospital Utrecht, Utrecht, The Netherlands

What happens with the aortic side branches? This has been the most common initial question vascular surgeons ask when confronted for the first time with endovascular exclusion of an abdominal aortic aneurysm (AAA). It is a very logical question if one realizes that with conventional AAA surgery the lumbar arteries and inferior mesenteric artery are ligated, whereas endovascular graft placement leaves all communications with the aneurysm sac intact. In theory, this situation is very similar to the anecdotal popliteal artery aneurysm that continues to grow from the back pressure of the geniculate arteries after being ligated above and below and bypassed.

The rapid dissemination of endovascular AAA surgery has led some individuals to believe that the side branch issue has been resolved or that it should be considered irrelevant. The opposite is true: after almost a decade of clinical application, it has become clear that incomplete exclusion of the aneurysm sac is, as G.W. White has commented, the Achilles' heel of endovascular AAA repair.

ENDOLEAKS

Incomplete AAA exclusion, or, more appropriately labeled, endoleak, is a condition associated with endoluminal vascular grafts, defined by the persistence of blood flow outside the lumen of the endoluminal graft but within an aneurysm sac or adjacent vascular segment being treated by the graft.[1] Endoleaks may appear immediately after an endograft placement (primary endoleak) or during follow-up (secondary endoleak). The reported incidence of primary endoleaks ranges from 7% to 49%.[2-7] Patent aortic side branches can only be considered part of the endoleak problem. Incomplete sealing at the attachment sites may also be responsible for blood flow outside the endovascular graft. Another source may be the body of the graft itself through inadequate connections in modular systems or defects in the fabric.

One of the most commonly used classifications of endoleaks has been proposed by White et al.[8] Attachment leaks are classified as type I endoleaks, and branch leaks are classified as type II. Recently, the same authors have added four other endoleak situations to this classification (Table 1).[9]

Although an attachment site leak or connection point leak can be considered a failure of the endovascular graft to attain its primary

TABLE 1.
Endoleak Classification by Source

Endoleak Type	Synonyms	Description
Type I	Perigraft EL or graft-related EL	Inadequate seal at proximal or distal graft attachment zones
Type II	Retrograde EL or non–graft-related EL	Persistent retrograde collateral blood flow into aneurysm sac retrograde from patent lumbar arteries or other collateral vessels
Type III	Fabric tear or modular disconnection	Leakage through a defect in the graft fabric or between segments of a modular graft
Type IV	Graft porosity	Minor blush of contrast on completion angiogram, emanating from blood diffusion across pores of a highly porous endograft
Undefined origin	—	Precise source of EL is unclear
Aneurysm sac pressure	Endopressure or endotension	No EL is demonstrated but the sac remains pressurized

Abbreviation: EL, endoleak.

goal (i.e., complete exclusion of the aneurysm), the presence of retrograde perfusion of the aneurysm sac by patent side branches is almost an inevitable consequence of the endovascular method. Using computed tomographic angiography (CTA) for selection of candidates for endovascular AAA repair, we noticed that all patients had one or several patent aortic side branches preoperatively.[10] This made us realize that, instead of focusing our attention on the question of why endoleaks develop in some patients, we should try to understand why not all patients are seen with endoleaks from patent side branches. This would also explain why the reported incidence of primary endoleaks is such a variable number. It would merely reflect the fact that some side branches need a little longer than others to stop perfusing the sac and that imaging methods are not 100% sensitive for detecting branch leaks.

CONSEQUENCES OF AN ENDOLEAK

The consequences of an endoleak are largely unknown. When designing management strategies for endoleaks, it must be realized that the primary goal of endovascular AAA repair is not to completely exclude the aneurysm sac but to prevent mortality (or early AAA repair–related morbidity and mortality) from a ruptured AAA.

Conventional AAA repair works because the diseased aortic segment prone to rupture is replaced by a prosthesis. Endovascular AAA repair essentially works in the same way, but there is a series of assumptions. Excluding the aneurysm from the aortic lumen will cause the remaining sac to thrombose. With this, the sac is depressurized, and, consequently, the sac will no longer be at risk for further growth and rupture. Conversely, endovascular repair fails if the sac does not completely thrombose (i.e., there is an endoleak) and, therefore, remains pressurized. This allows the sac to continue to grow and to be at risk for rupture.

If all these assumptions were true, it would make sense to always consider an endoleak as a treatment failure, and intervention would always be warranted. There are several reasons why it is not that simple.

THE UNPREDICTABILITY OF ENDOLEAKS

First, a large proportion of early endoleaks have been shown to spontaneously resolve. An endoleak can only be expected to stay open if there is sufficient blood flow or turbulence in the endoleak space or channel. If not, it will spontaneously thrombose within a short period of time. Most of these endoleaks will have sealed within the first few weeks after the operation, but it is not uncommon for an endoleak to seal even after 6 months. Although these spontaneously sealed endoleaks are observed very carefully, with respect to branch endoleaks, there is no obvious reason to believe that these may behave any differently from aortic side branches that thrombose spontaneously in the first minute after endograft placement. In the end, it is just a segment of thrombosed artery that separates the flow channel from the thrombus in the aneurysm sac. On the other hand, there is no reason to believe that the transmission of pressure through a large attachment leak is interrupted once the thrombus fills up the previously open endoleak space or channel. Nevertheless, it has been demonstrated that aneurysms can completely shrivel up after spontaneous thrombosis of branch leaks as well as large attachment site leaks.

Second, it is not uncommon for an aneurysm to maintain its original size or even grow in the months or years after endovascular AAA repair, even without a detectable endoleak. In these circumstances, the endoleak may have been missed by the studies used to detect it. Another explanation may be circumferential calcification of the aortic wall preventing the excluded sac from shrinking. However, the phenomenon also occurs in noncalcified walls. Most likely, some aneurysm sacs are fully thrombosed but not completely depressurized. Transmission of pressure into the sac can be main-

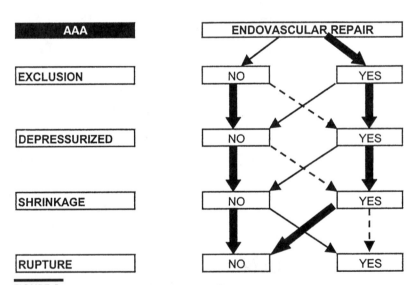

FIGURE 1.
Schematic representation of the uncertain relationships between the presence or absence of endoleaks (EXCLUSION), complete or incomplete depressurization (DEPRESSURIZED), size changes of the excluded sac (SHRINKAGE), and prevention of mortality from AAA rupture (RUPTURE). *Bold arrows* indicate likely consequence (50% to 100% chance), *light arrows* indicate possible consequence (5% to 50% chance), and *dashed arrows* indicate unlikely (but not impossible) consequence (0% to 5% chance). *Abbreviation: AAA*, abdominal aortic aneurysm.

tained through a communication between any arterial lumen and the thrombosed aneurysm sac. This pressure may originate from both aortic side branches and the main lumen (through inadequate endovascular seals or through defects in the endograft).

Third, even in the presence of endoleaks, aneurysms have been demonstrated to be capable of shrinking.

Figure 1 illustrates the aforementioned uncertainties in the relationships between the presence or absence of endoleaks, complete or incomplete depressurization, size changes of the excluded sac, and prevention of mortality from an AAA rupture.

The following examples illustrate the unpredictable nature of endoleaks.

CASE DESCRIPTIONS
CASE 1
A man, 75, with a 68-mm AAA received a 24- × 12-mm bifurcated endograft (Endovascular Technologies [EVT]/Guidant, Menlo Park, Calif). The procedure was uneventful, and completion angiography showed no signs of an endoleak. On postoperative CTA, an endoleak was found at the level of the native aortic bifurcation (Fig 2). A clear in- or outflow could not be visualized. The endoleak was accepted at first, but at 3 months, the AAA sac had increased in volume (285

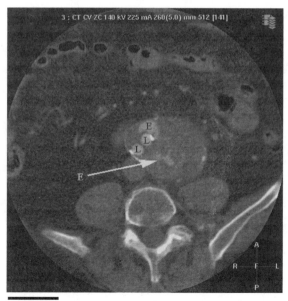

FIGURE 2.
Axial cut–plane of the CT angiographic scan of case 1, on day 1 postoperatively. *L* indicates the endograft limb, and *E* and *E arrow* indicate the endoleak.

mL vs. 262 mL postoperatively). Duplex examination suggested flow alongside the left iliac limb of the bifurcated endograft, originating from the left distal attachment system. An acute angle in the left common iliac artery together with heavy calcification was considered responsible for an inadequate distal left seal (Fig 3,A). In addition a significant endograft limb stenosis was found in this area.

A 15-mm Wallstent (Schneider, Bülach, Switzerland) was placed to straighten the limb and to treat the stenosis (Fig 3,B). Although flow around the left iliac limb could no longer be demonstrated via angiography, the aneurysm sac continued to show an endoleak, once again of unknown origin. We believed the Wallstent had turned the distal attachment site leak into a branch leak, and it was hoped that the remains of the endoleak would thrombose. Unfortunately, the endoleak persisted at 6 months postoperatively, and the sac continued to increase in volume (304 mL at 6 months and 327 mL at 12 months vs. 262 mL postoperatively) (Fig 4).

Although it would have been possible to approach the endoleak by means of endovascular intervention again, the patient chose to have the endograft removed. At conversion, pressures were measured in the aneurysm sac by putting a pressure needle into the aneurysm sac before clamping. It showed a damped pressure curve, but the mean pressure was almost identical to the mean systemic pressure (Fig 5).

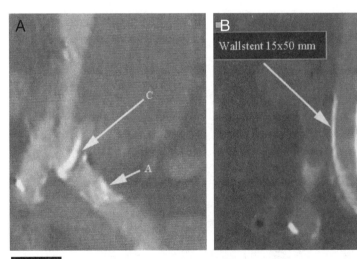

FIGURE 3.
Multiplanar CT angiographic reconstruction of left iliac limb of endoprosthesis of case 1, 3 months postoperatively: **A,** before a Wallstent is introduced—*C arrow* indicates calcified plaque and kink in the endograft limb and *A arrow* indicates distal attachment frame of left iliac endograft limb—and **B,** after placement of a 15- × 50-mm Wallstent—*C arrow* indicates the calcified lesion, now redressed. Note the Wallstent straightening out the kink in the iliac limb.

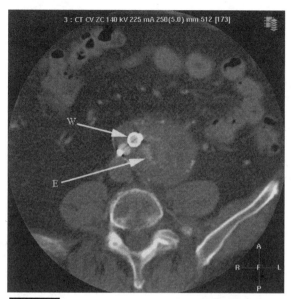

FIGURE 4.
Axial cut–plane of the CT angiographic scan of case 1, 3 months postoperatively after Wallstent placement. *W arrow* indicates the Wallstent and *E arrow* indicates the persistent endoleak.

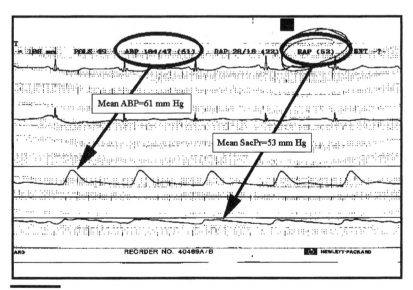

FIGURE 5.
Readings from pressure needle in aneurysm sac of case 1 at conversion 6 months after endograft placement. *Abbreviations: ABP,* arterial blood pressure (systemic); *RAP,* intrasac pressure (SacPr).

The pressure waves did not change when the clamps were placed proximal and distal to the aneurysm. The clamps were removed again, and the aneurysm sac was opened while the endograft was left intact. After removal of a large thrombus, a large, squirting middle sacral artery was detected. After this artery was ligated, the opened aneurysm sac was dry. The proximal and distal endovascular seals were adequate. At this point, we were ready to leave the situation as it was, but we respected the patient's wish to have the endograft replaced by a conventional graft. The postoperative course was complicated and protracted because of this patient's obesity, but he finally recovered well.

CASE 2
A man, 58, with a 74-mm AAA received a 26- × 13-mm bifurcated EVT graft. The procedure was uneventful, but on completion angiography, an endoleak at the proximal attachment site was seen (Fig 6). An additional balloon dilation of the proximal attachment system

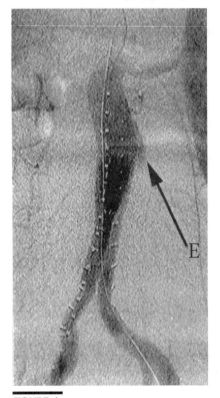

FIGURE 6.
Completion digital subtraction angiogram after endograft placement in case 2. *E arrow* indicates proximal attachment site endoleak.

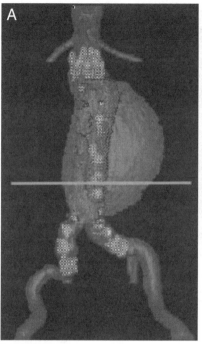

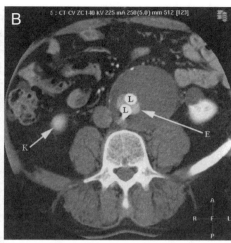

FIGURE 7.

CT angiogram of case 2, on day 2 postoperatively. **A**, three-dimensional recon-struction (surface display, anteroposterior view) with lumen, thrombus, endoleak, and endograft. **B**, axial cut–plane CT angiogram of the level indicated by *horizontal line* in **A**. *L*, endograft limb; *E arrow* indicates endoleak; *K arrow* indicates lower pole of right kidney.

was performed, but the endoleak persisted. The situation was accepted.

On postoperative CTA, an attachment site leak was found between the proximal and the right distal attachment systems (Fig 7). The patient was scheduled for a conversion as we thought this large attachment site leak would not resolve spontaneously. Preoperatively (11 days after endograft placement), a duplex study could not reproduce the endoleak. Subsequent CTA also failed to demonstrate the leak (Fig 8), and the conversion was canceled.

At follow-up, the excluded AAA continues to shrink, which indicates complete exclusion. The postoperative volume decreased from 297 mL at discharge to 157 mL at 3 months to 140 mL at 6 months and to 119 mL at 12 months.

CASE 3

A man, 71, with a 57-mm AAA received a 24- × 12-mm mono-iliac EVT graft in the left common iliac artery and an iliac–iliac

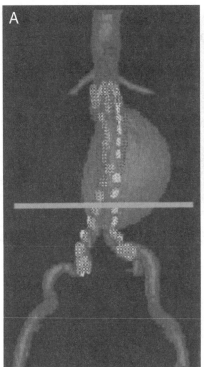
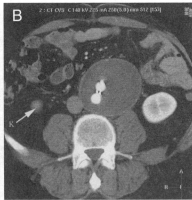

FIGURE 8.
CT angiogram of case 2, on day 11 postoperatively. **A**, three-dimensional reconstruction (surface display, anteroposterior view) with lumen, thrombus, and endograft. **B**, axial cut–plane CT angiogram of the level indicated by *horizontal line* in **A**. *K arrow* indicates lower pole of right kidney. No endoleak can be seen.

crossover graft (left to right) and ligation of the right common iliac artery proximal to the iliac bifurcation. The procedure was uneventful, and completion angiography showed no signs of an endoleak. It should be noted, however, that this angiogram was taken before recirculation of the right iliac artery. On postoperative CTA, a branch leak was found that was fed by an iliolumbar connection from the right hypogastric artery through the fourth lumbar artery into the aneurysm sac (Fig 9).

This situation was accepted initially, but at 6 months, the aneurysm volume had increased from 179 mL postoperatively to 222 mL. Therefore, the fourth lumbar artery was coil embolized via the right hypogastric artery all the way up into the aneurysm sac using a Tracker and Dasher-14 system (Target Therapeutics, Fremont, Ca; Boston Scientific, Natick, Mass) and a Tornado 6-2 mm coil (Cook, Inc., Bloomington, Ind) (Fig 10).

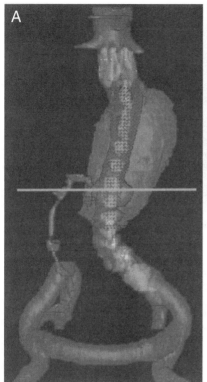
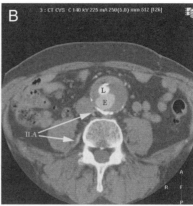

FIGURE 9.
CT angiogram of case 3, on day 1 postoperatively. **A**, three-dimensional reconstruction (surface display, anteroposterior view) with lumen, thrombus, endoleak and iliolumbar connection, and endograft. **B**, axial cut–plane CT angiogram of the level indicated by *horizontal line* in **A**. *L*, limb of mono-iliac endograft; *E*, endoleak; *ILA arrows* indicate iliolumbar artery.

At follow-up, the AAA continues to shrink, which indicates complete exclusion (189 mL at 6 months and 149 mL at 12 months).

CASE 4

A man, 67, with a 51-mm AAA received a 26- × 13-mm bifurcated EVT graft. The procedure was uneventful, and on completion angiography, no signs of an endoleak were seen. On postoperative CTA, a small branch endoleak was seen at the level of the native aortic bifurcation (Fig 11). This situation was accepted. Follow-up CT angiograms continued to demonstrate this branch endoleak, but the aneurysm volume decreased from 141 mL postoperatively to 101 mL at 6 months. The volume was again 101 mL at 12 months then decreased to 108 mL at 18 months (Fig 12). The situ-

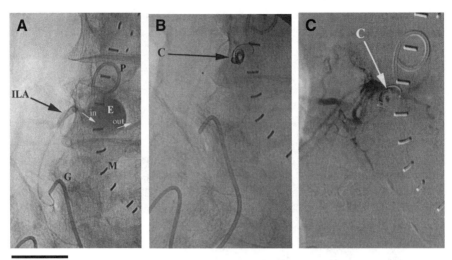

FIGURE 10.
Coil embolization of iliolumbar artery in case 3, 6 months postoperatively. **A**, superselective angiogram of iliolumbar artery (*ILA arrow*), showing entrance of contrast into the aneurysm sac (*in arrow*), filling the endoleak (*E*), and exiting through the contralateral lumbar artery (*out arrow*). *P*, pigtail catheter positioned in endograft; *M*, markers of endograft; *G*, guiding catheter (GlideCath; Terumo, Elkton, Md) advanced into the iliolumbar artery from the right hypogastric artery. **B**, Tornado coil (*C arrow*) deposited at the orifice of the ipsilateral fourth lumbar artery. **C**, superselective digital subtraction angiogram of iliolumbar artery showing no residual filling of the endoleak. *C arrow*, Tornado coil.

ation is still accepted but observed carefully; repeat CT angiograms are taken at 6-month intervals.

WHAT IS KNOWN ABOUT TREATING ENDOLEAKS?

There is a notorious lack of data on how to manage endoleaks. There are a few generally accepted guidelines based on large single-center experiences and multicenter registries (EUROSTAR).[11] Endoleaks that originate from an inadequate endovascular seal (endograft-to-artery attachment area or endograft-to-endograft connection point) or from defects in the endovascular graft (fabric tears) are generally considered treatment failures. These endoleaks connect to the main aortic lumen and maintain pressure in the aneurysm sac. Chances of spontaneous thrombosis are low, and if thrombosis occurs, pressure may still be transmitted via the thrombus into the sac. All case reports of AAA ruptures after endovascular repair that are available in the literature suggest this type of endoleak as the underlying cause of failure.[12-14] These attachment site or connection point endoleaks must be fixed using additional endovascular grafts or cuffs to seal the endoleak area. Filling these defects with endovascular coils has been described, but it frequently fails because of continued transmission of pressure through the area thrombosed via the coil. If all therapies fail to obliterate the endoleak and fail to induce aneurysm sac shrinkage, the patient is still considered at risk for aneurysm rupture, and conventional repair (conversion) is advised.

Although this approach to attachment site leaks is generally accepted, the cases described demonstrate the unpredictability of endoleaks. It would be more practical if it were possible to distinguish the harmful from the harmless endoleaks. On one hand, there are endoleaks (open or spontaneously thrombosed) that are capable of maintaining high pressure in the aneurysm sac to the extent that it continues to increase in size (the harmful type). Although it is currently unknown whether this puts the patient at the same risk for AAA rupture and death as before receiving the endovascular graft, it is clearly an uncomfortable situation for both the patient and the surgeon. On the other hand, there are endoleaks (open or thrombosed) that, for whatever reason, are

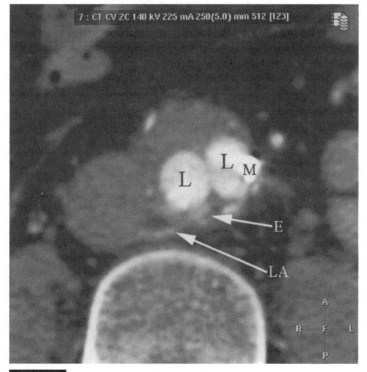

FIGURE 11.

Axial cut–plane of the CT angiographic scan of case 4, on day 1 postoperatively. *L,* limb of endograft; *M,* marker of endograft; *E arrow* indicates the endoleak; *LA arrow* indicates the connecting lumbar artery.

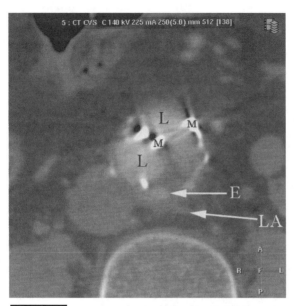

FIGURE 12.

Axial cut–plane of the CT angiographic scan of case 4, 12 months post-operatively. *L*, limb of endograft; *M*, marker of endograft; *E arrow* indicates the endoleak; *LA arrow* indicates the connecting lumbar artery.

incapable of maintaining pressure in the aneurysm (the harmless type).

Despite the availability of a large number of classifications of endoleaks based on time of detection, location, inflow, outflow, size, pressure, and involvement of branches, there is no accurate way of predicting whether an endoleak is going to be the harmful or harmless type.

Based on the aforementioned observations, we believe that not all endoleaks need treatment. It appears to be safe to wait a while (3 to 6 months) to allow the endoleak to identify itself as being either the harmless or harmful type, as determined by three-dimensional morphological features and the volume of the aneurysm sac during follow-up. Although it is also not known whether cessation of growth or even shrinkage is definite proof of a patient's protection against aneurysm rupture, it is currently the ultimate parameter of success.

FOLLOW-UP IMAGING

With our strategy, the imaging methods used for follow-up are of utmost importance. In most endovascular institutions, the maximum diameter of the aneurysm, as measured by CT or ultrasound, is used to gauge size changes after an endovascular repair.

Aneurysm morphological changes after an endovascular repair, however, are *volume* changes, and it is theoretically possible that volume changes occur without concomitant changes in the maximum diameter of the aneurysm. We have demonstrated cross-sectional CTA measurements (circumference cross-sectional area and maximum and minimum diameter) to be discordant with volume measurements in more than one third of follow-up cases. Often, volume shrinkage had been missed by cross-sectional measures; however, just as often, an increase in the volume of the aneurysm had been missed by cross-sectional measures. The latter, of course, is potentially dangerous if the decision to treat an endoleak is based on size changes.

We therefore advocate the use of volume measurements of the excluded aneurysm sac for follow-up. The problem with these volume measurements, however, is that it is a time-consuming effort (about 30 minutes per patient). Currently, there is no commercially available software package that can segment the aneurysm (lumen and thrombus) from the CTA data set automatically.

Our helical CTA acquisition protocol has been described elsewhere.[15] We use 140 mL of IV contrast with a scan delay of 40 seconds. The CTA data are transferred to an EasyVision Workstation (Philips, Best, The Netherlands). Cine mode viewing is used to detect endoleaks. This application of the workstation allows visualization of axial CT images in a movie-like fashion.[16] For volume measurements, the aortic lumen is segmented semiautomatically, and the aneurysm thrombus is segmented manually. After segmentation, the volume of the aneurysm is calculated between the level of the renal arteries and the level of the native aortic bifurcation.

OUR APPROACH TO THE ENDOLEAK PROBLEM

After endovascular graft placement, several completion angiographic runs are made focusing on the proximal and distal attachment areas intraoperatively. If an incomplete seal is detected, an attempt is made to repair it. The choice of therapy depends on the location of the endoleak, the type of device used, the availability of additional stents or cuffs, and the anatomy of the patient. Much effort is put into sealing an attachment site leak intraoperatively, but if this fails, the situation is accepted and not primarily converted to conventional repair.

If a branch leak appears on completion angiography, we do not attempt to close the branch at that time; we first verify, with several contrast runs, that it is not related to an obscure attachment site leak.

It has been suggested that branch endoleaks found intraoperatively should be sealed immediately (personal communication;

B.R. Hopkinson, January, 1999). Although this procedure has been demonstrated to decrease the number of endoleaks detected on postoperative CTA, it remains to be proven whether the leaks that are closed with these materials are indeed no longer pressurizing the sac and also whether the endoleaks that would have been left open if not treated would have posed any risk of continued aneurysm growth and rupture in the future. Preemptive coil embolization of all patent aortic side branches before endovascular grafting is unnecessary.[10,17]

The presence or absence of an endoleak on the postoperative (pre-discharge) CT angiogram on day 1 or 2 determines the frequency of follow up. If no endoleak is found, the next CTA is scheduled 6 months postoperatively. If an endoleak of any type is found on the first postoperative scan, CTA is repeated at 6 weeks (for scientific reasons only) and then at 3 and 6 months.

If the endoleak persists at or beyond 3 months, and, at the same time, the aneurysm volume increases, the situation must be remedied. Based on the endograft used, the type and location of the endoleak, and the condition of the patient, further therapy is selected. This can range from coil embolization of a lumbar artery or stent placement over an attachment area to laparoscopic lumbar artery clipping or conversion to conventional repair.

If an endoleak persists without an increase in volume, intervention is deferred until the 12-month follow-up CT angiogram. If the endoleak is still present at that time, intervention is scheduled.

If there is no detectable endoleak during follow up, regardless of whether the aneurysm was primarily excluded or the endoleak closed spontaneously or was closed by means of a secondary intervention, the volume of the aneurysm determines any further strategy. If the aneurysm volume decreases or if it does not change (without an endoleak), the endovascular repair is considered to be successful. After a few years of shrinkage, this process usually comes to a halt. If at any time the aneurysm sac increases in volume (with or without a detectable endoleak) on two consecutive CT angiograms, the patient is scheduled for contrast angiography with the intent of localizing the endoleak and, if possible, treating it by endovascular methods. If no endoleak can be found by any means, and the aneurysm sac continues to grow, conversion to conventional repair will be considered.

CONCLUSION

Although endoleaks have been labeled the "Achilles heel of endovascular surgery," it may well be that aneurysm volume changes after endovascular repair carry more predictive value for the long-term outcome of this procedure. Unfortunately, the first indication of a volume change cannot be given earlier than 3 to 6 months after endograft placement. In the first few days and months, the presence or absence and the type of endoleak may give both patient and surgeon an early indication of the success of the procedure. However, the unpredictability of endoleaks may lead to overtreatment if decisions are made too early. For an attachment site leak, it makes sense to initiate treatment early, as this type of endoleak is considered a primary treatment failure.

Branch leaks probably represent a much less dangerous situation in the short term. Other parameters such as the duration of the endoleak and aneurysm volume changes can help to improve the timing and selection of further intervention.

REFERENCES

1. White GH, Yu W, May J, et al: Endoleak as a complication of endoluminal grafting of abdominal aortic aneurysms: Classification, incidence, diagnosis, and management. *J Endovasc Surg* 4:152-168, 1997.
2. May J, White GH, Yu WY, et al: Repair of abdominal aortic aneurysms by the endoluminal method: Outcome in the first 100 patients. *Med J Aust* 165:549-551, 1996.
3. Parodi JC: Endovascular repair of aortic aneurysms, arteriovenous fistulas, and false aneurysms. *World J Surg* 20:655-663, 1996.
4. Moore WS, Rutherford RB: Transfemoral endovascular repair of abdominal aortic aneurysm: Results of the North American EVT phase 1 trial. EVT Investigators. *J Vasc Surg* 23:543-553, 1996.
5. Balm R, Eikelboom BC, May J, et al: Early experience with transfemoral endovascular aneurysm management (TEAM) in the treatment of aortic aneurysms. *Eur J Vasc Endovasc Surg* 11:214-220, 1996.
6. Chuter TAM, Risberg B, Hopkinson BR, et al: Clinical experience with a bifurcated endovascular graft for abdominal aortic aneurysm repair. *J Vasc Surg* 24:655-666, 1996.
7. Blum U, Voshage G, Lammer J, et al: Endoluminal stent-grafts for infrarenal abdominal aortic aneurysms. *N Engl J Med* 336:13-20, 1997.
8. White GH, May J, Waugh RC, et al: Type I and type II endoleaks: A more useful classification for reporting results of endoluminal AAA repair (letter). *J Endovasc Surg* 5:189-191, 1998.
9. White GH, May J, Waugh RC, et al: Type III and type IV endoleak: Toward a complete definition of blood flow in the sac after endoluminal AAA repair. *J Endovasc Surg* 5:305-309, 1998.
10. Broeders IA, Blankensteijn JD, Eikelboom BC: The role of infrarenal aortic side branches in the pathogenesis of endoleaks after endovascular aneurysm repair. *Eur J Vasc Endovasc Surg* 16:419-426, 1998.
11. Harris PL, Buth J, Mialhe C, et al: The need for clinical trials of endovascular abdominal aortic aneurysm stent-graft repair: The EUROSTAR project. *J Endovasc Surg* 4:72-77, 1997.
12. Torsello GB, Klenk E, Kasprzak B, et al: Rupture of abdominal aortic

aneurysm previously treated by endovascular stent graft. *J Vasc Surg* 28:184-187, 1998.

13. Alimi YS, Chakfe N, Rivoal E, et al: Rupture of an abdominal aortic aneurysm after endovascular graft placement and aneurysm size reduction. *J Vasc Surg* 28:178-183, 1998.
14. Lumsden AB, Allen RC, Chaikof EL, et al: Delayed rupture of aortic aneurysms following endovascular stent grafting. *Am J Surg* 170:174-178, 1995.
15. Broeders IAJM, Blankensteijn JD, Olree M, et al: Preoperative sizing of grafts for transfemoral endovascular aneurysm management: A prospective comparative study of spiral CT angiography, arteriography, and conventional CT imaging. *J Endovasc Surg* 4:252-261, 1997.
16. Balm R, Stokking R, Kaatee R, et al: Computed tomographic angiographic imaging of abdominal aortic aneurysms: Implications for transfemoral endovascular aneurysm management. *J Vasc Surg* 26:231-237, 1997.
17. Walker SR, Halliday K, Yusuf SW, et al: A study on the patency of the inferior mesenteric and lumbar arteries in the incidence of endoleak following endovascular repair of infrarenal aortic aneurysms. *Clin Radiol* 53:593-595, 1998.

CHAPTER 8

Laparoscopic Surgery for Abdominal Aortic Aneurysms

Joaquim J. Cerveira, M.D.
Vascular Fellow, Division of Vascular Surgery, Long Island Jewish Medical Center, New Hyde Park, New York

Jon R. Cohen, M.D.
Professor of Surgery, Albert Einstein School of Medicine, Bronx, New York; Chairman, Department of Surgery, Long Island Jewish Medical Center, New Hyde Park, New York

During the past 50 years, patients undergoing repair of abdominal aortic aneurysms (AAAs) have benefited from a progressive reduction in perioperative morbidity and mortality rates primarily because of improvements in anesthesia and surgical techniques.[1] With the use of current open techniques, clinical experience has shown that there is a mortality rate of less than 3% for elective AAA repair.[2] Long-term studies have demonstrated that conventional open repair is lasting, and it remains the standard of care.[3,4] Although conventional open repair is proven and reliable, exposure of the abdominal aorta requires a long midline or flank incision and extensive retroperitoneal dissection, which contribute to large fluid shifts, prolonged postoperative ileus, and significant postoperative pain and result in increased morbidity.[5,6]

Vascular surgeons are increasingly encountering older patients with severe co-morbid medical conditions, which can markedly increase operative mortality rates. Although therapies not involving resection, such as thrombosis of the aneurysm or aortic ligation with an axillofemoral bypass, have been suggested for use in high-risk patients, these techniques have not proven efficacious and have been widely abandoned because the procedures are not without risk and, even after transluminal thrombosis, rupture may still occur.[7]

A revolution of ideas and techniques has occurred in the vascular arena in response to the aging, high-risk patient. In 1991, the application of endovascular stents for infrarenal AAAs emerged as a minimally invasive alternative to conventional repair in high-risk patients undergoing surgery.[8] After initial success in animals, Parodi[8] introduced the concept of repairing an AAA with an endo-prosthesis introduced into the aorta through the femoral arteries. Success in applying this technique in humans was achieved using a device consisting of a compliant polyethylene terephthalate (Dacron) prosthesis attached to a Palmaz endoluminal stent. A review by Parodi[9] of his 4-year experience with the technique demonstrated that the procedure was associated with significant complications (e.g., graft migration, endoleaks, and thromboembolic events) and a substantial failure rate.

Since Parodi's initial experience, there has been substantial improvement in equipment, and there are now several endovascular grafts being studied for clinical use. There are, however, substantial limitations to, and concerns about, the endovascular technique, including control of endoleaks, continued dilatation of the aneurysm neck, delayed rupture of the aneurysm sac, and the need for lengthy follow-up and close surveillance. Nevertheless, investigational procedures continue to be developed in an attempt to establish safe, lasting techniques that result in minimal morbidity and mortality to the patient, improve cost reduction, and promote greater efficiency of health care provision.

USE OF LAPAROSCOPY IN VASCULAR SURGERY

The application of laparoscopic techniques to intra-abdominal vascular procedures is not new: laparoscopic exposure of the aorta during para-aortic lymph node dissection,[10] laparoscopic ligation of splenic artery aneurysms,[11] and aortic vascular reconstruction procedures using laparoscopic assistance have all been performed previously in humans.

In 1993, Dion and colleagues[12] reported the first aortobifemoral bypass using laparoscopic assistance. Laparoscopy was used to create a retroperitoneal cavity, similar to the balloon dissection technique used in laparoscopic preperitoneal hernia repair, which then allowed for dissection of the distal aorta and bilateral femoral arteries. The proximal aortic anastomosis was performed through a midline minilaparotomy without laparoscopic assistance. Standard groin incisions were then made, and the limbs of the graft were brought down to perform hand-sewn end-to-side anastomoses.

In an animal study, Ahn et al.[13] performed laparoscopic aortic bypass surgery on 16 pigs. Thirteen animals underwent transperitoneal dissection, and three underwent a retroperitoneal approach. Ten animals underwent laparoscopic aortofemoral bypasses; technical success was achieved in all. Vascular control was obtained by using Rumel tourniquets externalized through 5-mm trocar ports and an intraluminal balloon placed in the suprarenal aorta through the carotid artery as a backup system. The aortic anastomosis was performed using laparoscopic assistance and a combination of sutures and titanium clips. The femoral anastomoses were performed with the standard open technique. The mean operative time was 2.45 hours, and the mean blood loss was only 20 mL.

Continued modifications of laparoscopy, including use of a transperitoneal approach and gasless abdominal wall suspension and the development of bowel retractors, led to the first completely laparoscopic procedure involving a vascular anastomosis. By using a mechanical lift device, Berens and Herde[14] were able to use conventional vascular instruments for vessel clamping and suturing to perform two iliofemoral bypasses, one aortobifemoral bypass, and one aortoiliac endarterectomy. In this series, all patients were tolerating a regular diet by the second postoperative day, and all were discharged on the second or third postoperative day.

OPERATIVE TECHNIQUE

Our procedure of AAA repair using laparoscopic assistance is based on principles adopted from standard transabdominal laparoscopy as well as those of standard open endoaneurysmorrhaphy.

All patients referred for AAA repair have abdominal computerized axial tomography (CAT) scans. In addition, biplanar aortograms are obtained to evaluate the aorta and its branches for patency of collateral vessels (i.e., inferior mesenteric artery, median sacral artery, and lumbar arteries), to identify significant renal and other visceral arterial stenosis, and to adequately measure the length of the infrarenal aortic neck proximal to the aneurysm. The surgical risk is assessed in all patients after an appropriate medical evaluation and a required consultation.

Perioperative epidural analgesia is routinely used to reduce the need for narcotic pain control. A nasogastric tube and a Foley catheter are inserted to decompress the stomach and bladder. Hemodynamic monitoring may include radial artery, central venous, or pulmonary artery catheterization and transesophageal echocardiography. Continuous systemic and pulmonary arterial pressure readings are obtained as well as frequent cardiac outputs and indices, arterial blood gas levels, hemoglobin levels, platelet counts, serum chemical analyses, and coagulation profiles.

The patient is positioned supine with the legs straight and abducted. The operating surgeon is positioned between the patient's legs, the first assistant (camera holder) and third assistant stand to the left of the patient, and the second assistant (bowel retractor) stands to the right. All monitors and laparoscopic equipment are placed at the head of the patient (Fig 1). Initial intra-abdominal access is gained through a 1.0-cm midline supraumbilical incision. After the incision is made, a modified Glassman visceral retainer (Adept-Med) is placed directly into the peritoneal cavity. A 12-mm trocar is then inserted into the incision, and pneumoperitoneum is introduced to 15 mm Hg, using a warmed high-flow CO_2 insufflator. A 30-degree 10-mm laparoscope attached to a camera video system is introduced, and, under direct visualization,

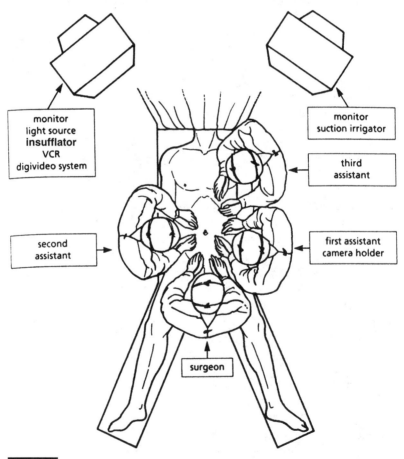

FIGURE 1.
Positions of operative team members.

an additional five 11-mm trocars are inserted (Fig 2). The patient is then placed in the Trendelenburg's position and rotated to the right. After the small bowel is retracted to the right and cephalad, the retroperitoneum is entered at the level of the duodenum with a combination of electrocautery and blunt dissection. Dissection continues until the neck of the aneurysm just inferior to the left renal vein is identified. At this point, approximately 75% of the circumference of the aorta, including the anterior surface and the lateral and medial surfaces down to the vertebral bodies, has been dissected with laparoscopic assistance. On completion of this task, the right and left common iliac vessels are dissected.

At completion of the laparoscopic dissection, all trocars are removed and an 8- to 10-cm minilaparotomy midline incision is

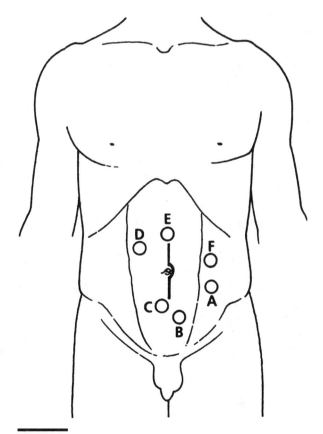

FIGURE 2.
Placement of trocars for aneurysm neck dissection and location of minilaparotomy. **A,** camera; **B,** dissector; **C,** dissector; **D,** bowel retractor; **E,** bowel retractor; **F,** suction/irrigation.

made at the level of the umbilicus. Through this incision, a Creech endoaneurysmorrhaphy is performed using standard instruments. The bowel is excluded with moist laparotomy pads, and an abdominal retractor is placed. Heparin (100 U/kg IV bolus) is then given, followed by occlusion of the iliac arteries with straight Fogarty clamps placed through trocar sites B and C (see Fig 2). The aneurysm neck is controlled with an aortic cross clamp introduced through trocar site E. The aneurysm is opened, and the ostia of bleeding collateral vessels are oversewn. A poly-tetrafluoroethylene (Gore-Tex; W.L. Gore, Flagstaff, Arizona) tube graft is sewn into place. The aortic wall is closed over the graft, and the retroperitoneum is closed over the aneurysm sac. All port sites are closed using single figure-of-eight absorbable sutures in the fascial layer. The minilaparotomy incision is closed in a single layer, and the skin incisions are closed with surgical staples.

Postoperative care is similar to the care required after open AAA repair, except that the recovery is more rapid. Patients will often be extubated within hours after surgery, will have earlier return of gastrointestinal function and tolerance of food in 2 to 3 days, and will often have shorter ICU and hospital stays.

CLINICAL EXPERIENCE

Investigation of alternative minimally-invasive approaches to aneurysmal surgery originated in the animal laboratory with a feasibility study to determine whether laparoscopic dissection and replacement of the intra-abdominal porcine aorta were possible.[15] Although the aorta was not calcified or aneurysmal, our initial studies revealed that laparoscopic dissection of the aorta was feasible but was associated with a significant learning curve. Twenty-one pigs underwent laparoscopic dissection of the abdominal aorta by a transabdominal approach and two pigs underwent laparoscopic dissection by a retroperitoneal approach. Fifteen grafts were successfully placed in the transperitoneal group, and one was successfully placed in the retroperitoneal group. Complications included injuries to the bladder, ureter, renal vein, inferior vena cava, aorta, and lumbar vessels. Operative times decreased from 6 to 2 hours, blood loss decreased from 1 L to 150 mL, and cross-clamp time decreased from 60 to 20 minutes by the conclusion of the study.

On the basis of the initial encouraging results of this feasibility study, we undertook a survival study to compare the hemodynamic and postoperative results of pigs undergoing open vs. laparoscopic replacement of the abdominal aorta.[16] Twenty pigs were divided into four groups. Aortic replacement was accomplished by (1) an open hand-sewn graft, (2) open insertion of a cuffed graft, (3) laparoscopic assistance, or (4) total laparoscopic insertion of a cuffed graft. The cuffed graft is similar in concept to the grafts used for the treatment of thoracic aortic dissection. The aorta was replaced in all animals, and no intraoperative deaths occurred. There were no differences between groups in blood loss, fluid requirement, temperature, and urine output. Except for the cardiac index, there were no differences in systemic and pulmonary hemodynamics. The two laparoscopic groups maintained a higher cardiac index during cross clamping of the aorta. The cross-clamp time was the longest in the group in which a laparoscope was used and the graft was sewn in through a small minilaparotomy. The operative time for the laparoscopic group was longer than that for the open control group. However, the longer operative time did not result in more profound hypothermia, most likely because of the use of a heated insufflator and smaller incisions.

Information learned in the animal laboratory was applied to human AAA repair using laparoscopic assistance.[17] With institutional review board approval, we carefully selected patients with infrarenal AAAs requiring tube grafts and with no contraindications for laparoscopy. Our operative goals were to dissect the neck of the aneurysm and both iliac arteries using laparoscopic assistance, then, through a minilaparotomy, cross clamp the aorta, and repair the aneurysm using a conventional open Creech technique.[4] To date, a preliminary study of 20 patients has been completed.[18] In 18 patients, the dissection was successfully completed; conversion to a standard open incision was necessary because of inadequate port placement in patient 1 and because of multiple adhesions caused by a previous hysterectomy in patient 13. Several factors may lead to a conversion from an AAA repair with laparoscopic assistance to an open AAA repair. The presence of dense adhesions and the lack of adequate hemostasis are two common reasons. Other possible reasons include poor exposure and the presence of an inflammatory aneurysm.

In the animal studies, the dissection ports were placed in the lower abdomen. Although these port positions were ideal for the iliac dissection, they were too low to get over the hump of the aneurysm and reach the neck. Modifications in the trocar location resulted in successful laparoscopic dissection of the neck of the aorta and the iliac vessels.

In the immediate postoperative period, there were three minor complications, all of which were unrelated to the laparoscopy. In one patient, a superficial wound infection developed, requiring 2 additional days of IV antibiotics. In another patient, a mild case of rhabdomyolysis developed after plaque emboli from an iliac cross clamp occurred; the case was successfully treated by IV hydration. In the third patient, who had undergone an uncomplicated AAA repair with laparoscopic assistance 8 days after undergoing combined coronary artery bypass grafting and aortic and mitral valve replacements, a pericardial effusion developed that required a pericardial window. There was a single major complication of postoperative left-sided colonic ischemia. The patient underwent a Hartmann's procedure and subsequently became ventilator dependent.

Operative times averaged 4.09 ± 0.92 hours, which were longer than the standard times of 3 to 3.5 hours for open approaches. The time used for laparoscopy, which accounted for about 40% of the total operative time, was 1.40 ± 0.45 hours. With increased experience, we decreased this operative time to less than 1 hour (Fig 3). Most patients were extubated within hours after completion of the procedure (Fig 4). The mean duration of nasogastric tube suctioning was 1.3 ± 0.7 days, and 14 of the 18 patients tolerated a clear liquid diet by the second postoperative day (Fig 5). The mean ICU stay was 2.2 ± 0.9 days, and the mean length of hospitalization was 5.8 ± 1.6 days (Figs 6 and 7). The patients appeared to return to their preoperative status with-

TOTAL OPERATIVE TIME

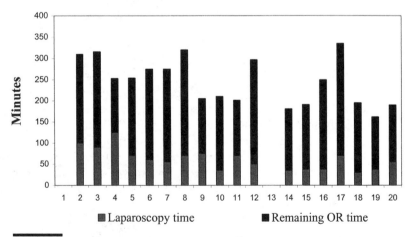

FIGURE 3.
Laparoscopic and total operating room (OR) times excluding patients whose procedures were converted to open abdominal aortic aneurysm repair.

TIME TO EXTUBATION

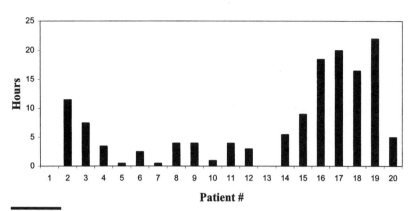

FIGURE 4.
Hours to extubation.

GI FUNCTION

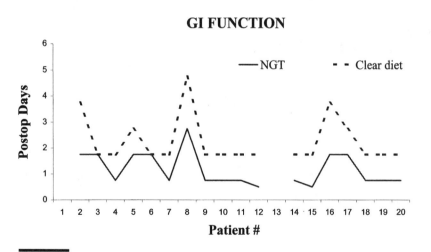

FIGURE 5.
Duration of NGT suction and interval to tolerating a clear liquid diet. *Abbreviations: GI,* gastrointestinal; *NGT,* nasogastric tube.

in 2 to 3 weeks after the operation in terms of their energy levels, the levels of their activity, and their appetites. There were no deaths in this study.

ICU STAY

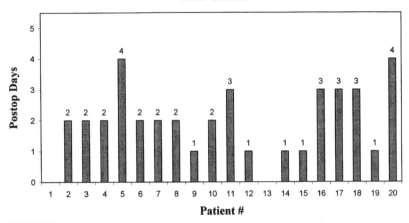

HOSPITAL STAY

FIGURE 6.
Duration of postoperative recovery in ICU.

HOSPITAL STAY

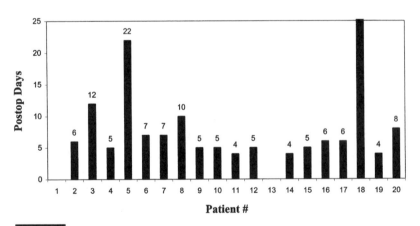

FIGURE 7.
Length of hospitalization.

LESSONS LEARNED

After completion of our initial feasibility study, we investigated transperitoneal and retroperitoneal approaches to the abdominal aorta. Our animal laboratory experience identified a significant difficulty in maintaining an adequately insufflated cavity in the retroperitoneum, especially after a tear in the peritoneum. Small tears may be sutured using laparoscopic assistance, but large rents nearly always require conversion to an open procedure. In addition, control of the right iliac artery can be difficult with the retroperitoneal exposure, especially in cases of large aneurysms. The main advantage of the retroperitoneal approach is the total avoidance of direct bowel contact. However, with the development of the modified visceral retractor, the bowel is easily retracted.

Injuries to adjacent organs can be a potential morbid, if not lethal, complication. The bladder, the ureters and kidneys, the gonadal and renal veins, the inferior vena cava, the sympathetic chain, of which all are located within the operative field especially close to the aorta and iliac arteries, are subject to injury unless they are clearly identified. Our initial ten dissections in the porcine model resulted in six injuries; however, after gaining experience with the anatomy and the technique, no injuries were observed with the last ten procedures performed. Of our first 20 procedures in patients, no adjacent organ injuries have been observed. Injuries are less common as the surgeon gains technical skill and can be avoided by clearly recognizing anatomical structures and their locations as each maneuver is performed.

Control of bleeding is probably the main concern that limits the adoption of AAA repair using laparoscopic assistance. Bleeding may occur at any stage of the operation; however, we have observed that, as with the standard open technique, it is most likely to be encountered during the exposure and ligation of lumbar vessels. Others have reported the laparoscopic identification, dissection, and division of lumbar vessels during AAA repair; however, we do not believe that the risk of uncontrolled bleeding with the need for immediate conversion to an open procedure merits this.[19] Our modification of performing a minilaparotomy after laparoscopic dissection is an attempt to directly control bleeding and to facilitate placement of the vascular graft. Arterial bleeding can often be managed with temporary direct pressure followed by suture ligation or endoclip application. A concern about air emboli while using carbon dioxide insufflation for vascular surgery has also been voiced; however, Dion and associates[20] have shown that, with a 1-cm phlebotomy in the inferior vena cava, pigs do not sustain pulmonary emboli.

FUTURE DEVELOPMENTS

At present, we have used laparoscopy in AAA repairs of aneurysms that required tube grafts, but, as Edoga and associates[19] have reported, and as the previous work of Dion et al., Ahn et al.,[13] and others have demonstrated, iliac disease should not be a contraindication. The use of laparoscopy in placing a bifurcated graft for an AAA is a natural progressive step in the joining of our current skills and those demonstrated for aortoiliac disease.

Another problem that must be tackled is controlling lumbar bleeding when using the transperitoneal approach. In many cases, the lumbar vessels are inaccessible because of concerns about causing significant damage to the retroperitoneal aortic venous plexus and showering emboli from the atherosclerotic aorta. Current stapling devices frequently cannot occlude patent collateral vessels in the opened, atherosclerotic aorta, but as instrumentation is developed, the significant bleeding occasionally seen from patent lumbar vessels will be minimized.

Currently, no completely laparoscopic AAA repair has been reported. The difficulties include the control of bleeding, the technical difficulties of suturing vascular grafts to a diseased aorta and distal vessels using laparoscopic assistance, and the prolonged aortic clamp time required. Zegdi et al.[21] recently reported the investigational use of a sutureless prosthesis for aortic replacement. A polyethylene terephthalate graft with an inverted collar was inserted into the aortic lumen, then fixed circumferentially to the arterial wall with titanium clips. No anastomotic leak was noted during sustained periods of hypertension, and blood loss was minimal during the procedures. With current secure laparoscopic vascular clamps and the development of sutureless prosthetic materials, the need for a minilaparotomy should be obviated and a totally laparoscopic procedure should evolve.

Currently, the lower size limit for aneurysms in aneurysm repair, in most series, is approximately 5.0 cm.[1] Given current mortality rates, it is generally believed that open surgery for aneurysms less than 5.0 cm is not beneficial because of an adverse risk–benefit ratio.[22] If total laparoscopic AAA repair can be performed with minimal morbidity and mortality, operations on smaller aneurysms may well be considered appropriate, particularly because of the improved anatomical exposure using laparoscopy.

CONCLUSION

Since the first description of AAAs by the 16th century anatomist Vesalius, the history of this disease has reflected the remarkable progress of vascular surgery. The present-day vascular surgeon is supplied with a technically evolving armamentarium that has gone from initial attempts at ligation and sclerosis to the recent advances of endovascular and laparoscopic repair. None of these procedures is mutually exclusive. Currently, great interest lies in the use of laparoscopy to provide extraluminal control at the neck of aneurysms for the purpose of working with endoluminal grafts and controlling collateral vessel endoleaks.

We believe that laparoscopic vascular surgery must not be introduced into the clinical arena based on the unique assumption that it is a feasible technique. Clearly, it is a technically challenging procedure with a steep learning curve, and it requires specialized instrumentation and sophisticated laparoscopic suturing capabilities. However, we believe that with continued investigation including prospective randomized trials, laparoscopic treatment of aortic aneurysms may become a standard option for high-risk patients.

REFERENCES

1. Ernst CB: Abdominal aortic aneurysm. *N Engl J Med* 328:1167-1172, 1993.
2. Whittemore AD, Clowes AW, Hechtman HB, et al: Aortic aneurysm repair: Reduced operative mortality associated with maintenance of optimal cardiac performance. *Ann Surg* 192:414-421, 1980.
3. Crawford ES, Saleh SA, Babb JW, et al: Infrarenal abdominal aortic aneurysm: Factors influencing survival after operation over a 25-year period. *Ann Surg* 193:699-706, 1981.
4. Creech O Jr: Endoaneurysmorrhaphy and treatment of aortic aneurysm. *Ann Surg* 164:935-946, 1966.
5. Cambria RP, Brewster DC, Abbott WM, et al: Transperitoneal versus retroperitoneal approach for aortic reconstruction: A randomized prospective study. *J Vasc Surg* 11:314-317, 1990.
6. Paty PSK, Darling RC III, Chang BB, et al: A prospective randomized study comparing exclusion technique and endoaneurysmorrhaphy for treatment of infrarenal aortic aneurysm. *J Vasc Surg* 25:442-445, 1997.
7. Resnikoff M, Darling RC, Chang BB, et al: Fate of the excluded abdominal aortic aneurysm sac: Long-term follow-up of 831 patients. *J Vasc Surg* 24:851-855, 1996.
8. Parodi JC, Palmaz JC, Barone HD: Transfemoral intraluminal graft implantation for abdominal aortic aneurysms. *Ann Vasc Surg* 5:491-499, 1991.
9. Parodi JC: Endovascular repair of abdominal aortic aneurysms and other arterial lesions. *J Vasc Surg* 21:549-557, 1995.
10. Childers JM, Surwit EA: Laparoscopic para-aortic lymph node biopsy for diagnosis of a non-Hodgkin's lymphoma. *Surg Laparosc Endosc* 2:139-142, 1992.
11. Hashizume M, Ohta M, Ueno K, et al: Laparoscopic ligation of splenic artery aneurysm. *Surgery* 113:352-354, 1993.
12. Dion YM, Katkhouda N, Rouleau C, et al: Laparoscopy-assisted aorto-bifemoral bypass. *Surg Laparosc Endosc* 3:425-429, 1993.
13. Ahn SS, Clem MF, Braithwaite BD, et al: Laparoscopic aortofemoral bypass. *Ann Surg* 222:677-683, 1995.
14. Berens ES, Herde JR: Laparoscopic vascular surgery: Four case reports. *J Vasc Surg* 22:73-79, 1995.
15. Chen MHM, Murphy EA, Levison J, et al: Laparoscopic aortic replace-

ment in the porcine model: A feasibility study in preparation for laparoscopically assisted abdominal aortic aneurysm repair in humans. *J Am Coll Surg* 183:126-132, 1996.

16. D'Angelo AJ, Chen MHM, Murphy EA, et al: Comparison of laparoscopic and open abdominal aortic replacement in the porcine model. *Surg Endosc* 10:228A, 1996.

17. Chen MHM, Murphy EA, Halpern V, et al: Laparoscopic-assisted abdominal aortic aneurysm repair. *Surg Endosc* 9:905-907, 1995.

18. Kline RG, D'Angelo AJ, Chen MHM, et al: Laparoscopically assisted abdominal aortic aneurysm repair: First 20 cases. *J Vasc Surg* 27:81-88, 1998.

19. Edoga JK, Asagarian K, Singh D, et al: Laparoscopic surgery for abdominal aortic aneurysms: Technical elements of the procedure and a preliminary report of the first 22 patients. *Surg Endosc* 12:1064-1072, 1998.

20. Dion YM, Levesque C, Doillon CJ: Experimental carbon dioxide pulmonary embolization after vena cava laceration under pneumoperitoneum. *Surg Endosc* 9:1065-1069, 1995.

21. Zegdi R, Martinod E, Fabre O, et al: A new vascular prosthesis: Potential interests in mini-invasive aortic surgery (abstract 3), in *Proceedings of Angio-Techniques: Alternatives and Techniques in Vascular Diseases*. Marseille, France, 1999, pp 38-44.

22. Nevitt MP, Ballard DJ, Hallett JW: Prognosis of abdominal aortic aneurysms: A population-based study. *N Engl J Med* 321:1009-1014, 1989.

PART III
Infrainguinal Disease

C HAPTER 9

Endovascular In Situ Bypass

David Rosenthal, M.D.
Clinical Professor of Surgery, Medical College of Georgia, Georgia Baptist
Medical Center, Atlanta, Georgia

In 1962, Karl Viktor Hall reported the first successful femoropopliteal in situ saphenous vein bypass.[1] Since this initial report, surgeons have attempted to make the in situ saphenous vein bypass a less invasive operation while simplifying the two principal technical components of the operation: (1) rendering the saphenous vein valves incompetent and (2) occluding the venous side branches. For this to be accomplished, however, it is often necessary to make a long incision along the length of the leg over the course of the saphenous vein, which can be fraught with hazard, especially in the patient with diabetes, in whom wound complications can be devastating.

A technique using an angioscope has been developed that allows the surgeon to perform a valvulotomy and to occlude venous side branches from within the saphenous vein: the minimally invasive endovascular in situ vein bypass (EISB). After several generations of change and refinement of the endovascular instrumentation and technique of operation, today the EISB is performed using the Fogarty valvulotome and an angioscopic-guided Side Branch Occlusion System (Baxter Vascular, Irvine, Calif) that is elegant in its simplicity and user friendly.

The component parts of the system are the retrograde Fogarty valvulotome, which houses an irrigating catheter (for a heparin–papaverine–saline flush) and is introduced from the distal saphenous vein (Fig 1). The Side Branch Occlusion System is introduced from the proximal saphenous vein and consists of a movable angioscope and the coil delivery catheter, which contains a preloaded Gianturco occlusion coil (Target Therapeutics, San Jose, Calif) and guide wire. This new system allows the valvuloto-

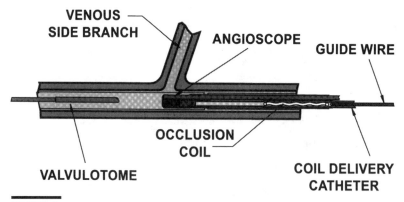

FIGURE 1.
Valvulotome and Side Branch Occlusion System. (Courtesy of Rosenthal
D: Angioscopy in vascular surgery. *Cardivasc Surg* 5(3):245-255, 1997.
With permission from Elsevier Science.)

my and side branch occlusion to be performed with a single pass
down the saphenous vein.

TECHNIQUE OF OPERATION
VALVULOTOMY

Before valvulotomy, the angioscope is placed in the extended position, which allows visualization of the vein lumen in a 360-degree
circumferential fashion (Fig 2). At this point, the valvulotome cutting blades are kept retracted to minimize any potential for intimal
trauma. When a set of valve leaflets are identified, the cutting
blade is extended and a valve leaflet is engaged (Fig 3). With gentle traction on the valvulotome, the surgeon performs the valvulo-

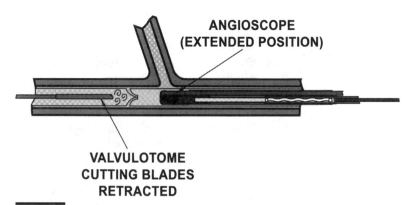

FIGURE 2.
Angioscope is in extended position, and valvulotome cutting blade is
retracted.

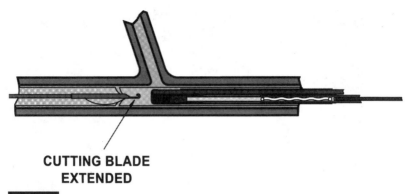

**CUTTING BLADE
EXTENDED**

FIGURE 3.
Valvulotome cutting blade is extended, and the valve leaflet is engaged.

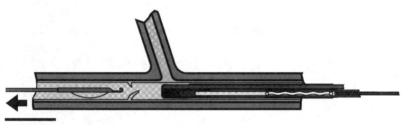

FIGURE 4.
Valvulotomy of one leaflet is completed.

tomy under direct angioscopic surveillance in two planes (Fig 4), and the valvulotome cutting blade is then retracted.

SIDE BRANCH OCCLUSION

Most major side branches are located at the site of vein valves, so side branch occlusion can be immediately performed after a valvulotomy. (Note: There is no consistent order to the valvulotomy and side branch occlusion procedures. Either maneuver may be performed first, it is merely the surgeon's discretion.) When a side branch is visualized (Fig 5), the angioscope is placed into the retracted position, which allows better visualization of the side branch orifice (Fig 6).

The coil delivery catheter, which contains the occlusion coil and guide wire, is then guided into the side branch (Fig 7); the guide wire is advanced, and a coil is deployed from the delivery catheter (Fig 8) into the venous side branch; and the side branch is embolized (Fig 9).

With this new technique, valvulotomy and side branch occlusion may be easily and safely performed with a single pass down the saphenous vein through two incisions (Figs 10 and 11).

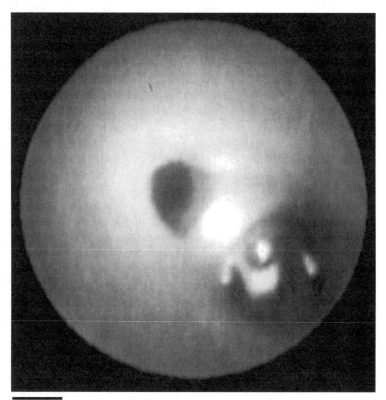

FIGURE 5.
Angioscopic image of side branch orifice. *Note*: valvulotome is distal in vein.

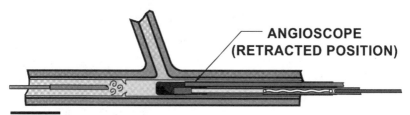

FIGURE 6.
Angioscope is in retracted position.

An ongoing multicenter study was initiated using this angioscopic technique. A total of 102 minimally invasive EISB procedures (27 femorodistal popliteal and 75 femorocrural) and 104 conventional "open" in situ bypasses have been done. Current results demonstrate that 60 minimally invasive bypasses were performed through two incisions, 16 required a third incision, and 28 operations required four or more incisions. The extra incisions were necessary to ligate large venous side branches (larger than 5

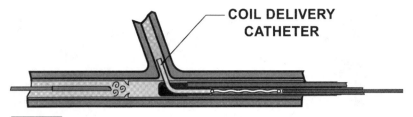

FIGURE 7.
The coil delivery catheter containing an occlusion coil is guided into the side branch.

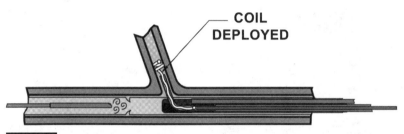

FIGURE 8.
Gianturco coil is deployed from coil delivery catheter.

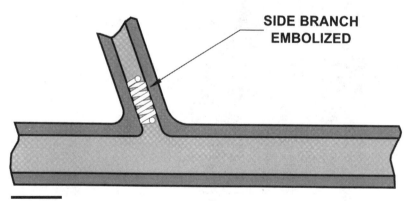

FIGURE 9.
Embolized side branch.

mm in diameter) or missed arteriovenous fistulas. On average, 6.2 side branches have been embolized per operation; more distal bypasses obviously require more side branch occlusions. There were 6 (5.8%) wound complications in the EISB group vs. 19 (18.6%) in the conventional group. The mean hospital length of stay (LOS) for the patients undergoing EISB has been 2.8 days vs. 6.9 days for the patients undergoing the conventional operation. The potential for wound complications and the hospital LOS have

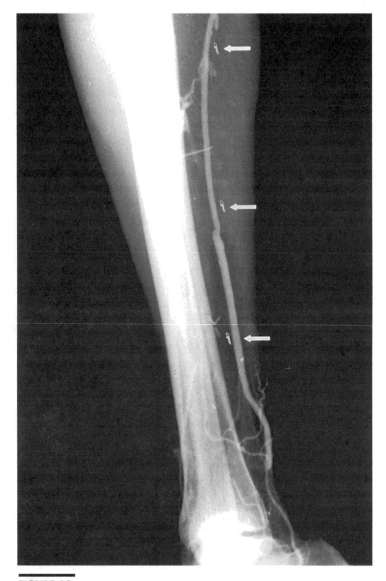

FIGURE 10.
Completion arteriogram demonstrates a patent endovascular femoroposterior tibial in situ bypass. *Note*: coil occluded vein side branches.

been greatly reduced with the minimally invasive EISB bypass because the need for an incision along the length of the leg is avoided. The primary bypass graft patency at 36 months was 72% in the EISB group and 75% in the conventional group ($P = 0.12$), and the secondary patency rate was 80% and 83%, respectively (P

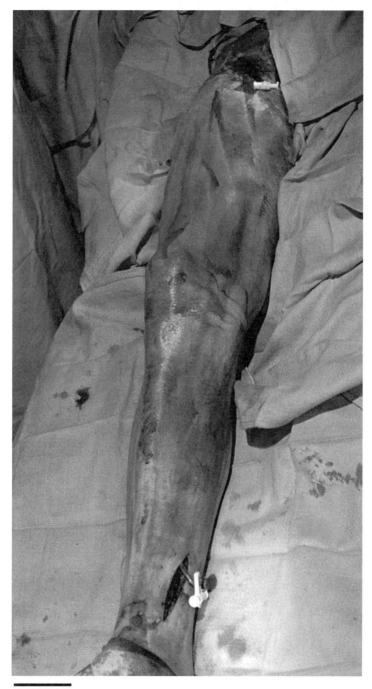

FIGURE 11.
Endovascular femoroposterior tibial bypass performed through two incisions.

= 0.05). The limb salvage rate was 88% for the EISB group and 91% for the conventional in situ group. The primary patency rates of the EISB grafts at 36 months (72%) are comparable with those found in the excellent reports by Leather et al.[2] (79%) and Donaldson et al.[3] (70%) using the classic open in situ operation, which serves as the bench mark against which in situ bypass data must be compared (Fig 12).

One area of concern was the noted drop in patency within the first 6 months in the EISB grafts. This is attributed to the learning curve of the operation, which has two components: (1) learning a new technique of operation and the instrumentation itself and (2) learning to judge which patients are appropriate for this technique. Early in the multicenter study, it is likely that we were too aggressive, wanting to do all operations with the endovascular technique, and that we pushed the instrumentation excessively. It is now apparent that in small veins—those less than 2.5 to 3.0 mm in diameter after dilation—we likely traumatized the vein, which led to early graft failures.

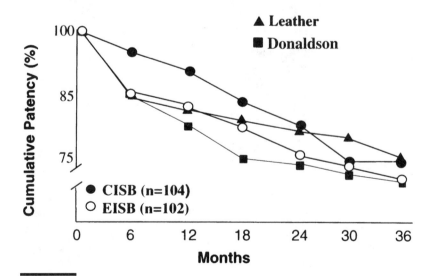

FIGURE 12.

Primary patency rates at 36 months' follow-up. *Abbreviations: EISB,* endovascular in situ vein bypass; *CISB,* conventional in situ bypass.[12]

Reservation Card for Advances

Yes! I would like my own copy of *Advances in Vascular Surgery*® at the price of **$83.00** (**$92.00** outside the U.S.) plus sales tax, postage, and handling. Please begin my subscription with the current edition according to the terms described below.* I understand that I will have 30 days to examine each annual edition.

Name _____

Address _____

City _____ State _____ ZIP _____

Method of Payment

Check (in U.S. dollars, drawn on a U.S. bank, payable to *Advances in Vascular Surgery*®)

❑ VISA   ❑ MasterCard   ❑ Discover   ❑ AmEx   ❑ Bill me

Card number _____ Exp. date: _____

Signature _____

Prices are subject to change without notice.   PMC-377

Subscribe to the related journal in your field!

Yes! Begin my one-year subscription to *Journal of Vascular Surgery* (12 issues).

Name _____

Institution _____

Address _____

City _____ State _____

ZIP/PC _____ Country _____

Specialty _____
(Students/residents, please list Institution)

Subscription prices (through 9/30/99)

		USA	Canada*	Int'l
Individuals	❑	$161.00	$212.93	$199.00
Institutions	❑	306.00	368.08	344.00
Students, residents	❑	83.00	129.47	121.00

Method of payment

Enclose payment (check or credit card number) and we'll send an extra issue FREE!

❑ Check (in U.S. dollars, drawn on a U.S. bank, and payable to *Journal of Vascular Surgery*)

❑ VISA   ❑ MasterCard   ❑ Discover
❑ AmEx   ❑ Bill me   Exp. date_____

Card #_____

Signature _____

*Includes Canadian GST

Individual/student subscriptions must be in the name of, billed to, and paid for by the individual.

Airmail rates available upon request.
Prices subject to change without notice.

                                        J024991YC

---

*Your Advances service guarantee:

When you subscribe to *Advances*, you will receive advance notice of future annual volumes about two months before publication. To receive the new edition, you need do nothing—we'll send you the new volume as soon as it is available. If you want to discontinue, the advance notice allows you time to notify us of your decision. If you are not completely satisfied, you have 30 days to return any *Advances*.

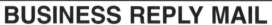

BUSINESS REPLY MAIL
FIRST-CLASS MAIL   PERMIT NO 135   ST LOUIS MO

POSTAGE WILL BE PAID BY ADDRESSEE

SUBSCRIPTION SERVICES
MOSBY, INC.
11830 WESTLINE INDUSTRIAL DRIVE
ST. LOUIS   MO 63146-9988

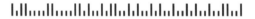

BUSINESS REPLY MAIL
FIRST-CLASS MAIL   PERMIT NO 135   ST LOUIS MO

POSTAGE WILL BE PAID BY ADDRESSEE

SUBSCRIPTION SERVICES
MOSBY, INC.
11830 WESTLINE INDUSTRIAL DRIVE
ST. LOUIS   MO 63146-9988

NO POSTAGE
NECESSARY
IF MAILED
IN THE
UNITED STATES

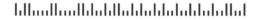

Want to speed up the process?

**To order a *Year Book* or *Advances*,
you also may call 1-800-426-4545**

**To subscribe to a journal today,
call toll-free in the U.S.:
1-800-453-4351
or fax 314-432-1158
Outside the U.S., call: 314-453-4351**

Visit us at: *www.mosby.com/periodicals*

Mosby, Inc.
Subscription Services
11830 Westline Industrial Drive
St. Louis, MO   63146 U.S.A.

 Mosby

Infrainguinal in situ saphenous vein bypass remains one of the most challenging operations facing the vascular surgeon today. Patients undergoing this procedure often have complicated medical and surgical problems, and the rising health care costs in the United States today have made minimally invasive operations most attractive. Gupta and Veith[4] demonstrated the inadequacy of diagnosis-related group (DRG) reimbursement for limb salvage arterial reconstructions. Their study evaluated the cost of 209 patients in ten centers who underwent saphenous vein bypasses for limb salvage. The net reimbursement to the hospital for each patient was a loss of $5,616, or a total study loss of $1,382,744! The basic cause of this problem was the protracted mean LOS (18.8 days) (Gupta, personal communication May, 1993), which, in large part, was due to the morbidity associated with an incision along the length of the leg.

In this cost-conscious health care era, the following concern must be addressed: is the minimally invasive EISB procedure cost-effective? The cost of the endovascular instrumentation is $2,000, and surgeons have appropriately voiced concern about justifying this additional cost to their hospital administrations. It is of interest to look at this through the perspective of DRG reimbursement and what it means to the hospital (Table 1). The 1996 Health Care Financing Administration data on 3,045 operative payments for International Classification of Diseases-ninth revision (ICD-9) code 440.31 (i.e., lower extremity arterial revascularization with saphenous vein) are quite shocking. The data demonstrate a mean LOS of 7.5 days, and if we take the mean charges less the mean payments, the result is a net loss of $12,000 per patient or a loss to hospitals of more than $36 million in 1996! In the ongoing multicenter study, the conventional group demonstrated a mean LOS that was reduced; therefore, the net loss in dollars per patient was

TABLE 1.

Hospital LOS and Cost Data

	HCFA (1996)	**CISB**	**EISB**
LOS (days)	7.5	5.9	2.8
Charges ($)	23,000	21,700	16,300
Payment ($)	11,000	12,400	12,400
Net ($)	−12,000	−9,300	−3,900

Abbreviations: LOS, length of stay; *HCFA,* Health Care Financing Administration; *CISB,* conventional in situ bypass; *EISB,* endovascular in situ vein bypass.

lower. For the EISB group, however, the mean LOS was decreased by half and the net loss was reduced by two thirds, thus narrowing the gap toward profitability for the hospital. It appears, therefore, that not only does the patient benefit by a less invasive operation but also the expense of the instrumentation can be justified to the hospital administration.

The limitations of the minimally invasive in situ vein bypass are, foremost, the size and quality of the saphenous vein. In veins less than 3 mm in diameter, it may be too difficult to maneuver the catheter into venous side branches without causing intimal injury. In general, venous side branches at or above the knee, because they are larger, are most easily occluded, but endovascular occlusion of all saphenous vein side branches may not be possible in each vein graft. The technique, however, continues to evolve, and as refinement of the technique and catheter design continue and operator experience increases, it is hoped that these limitations will be overcome.[5]

If the minimally invasive EISB long-term patency rates remain similar to classic in situ bypass patency rates, the benefits we will see of decreased hospital LOS, reduced wound-related complications, shortened recuperation, and, therefore, increased health care savings indicate that this minimally invasive endovascular technique will be an appropriate adjunct for the patient who requires an in situ saphenous vein bypass.

REFERENCES

1. Hall KV: The great saphenous vein used in-situ as an arterial shunt after extirpation of the vein valves. *Surgery* 51:492-495, 1962.
2. Leather RP, Shah DJ, Chang BB: Resurrection of the in situ saphenous vein bypass 1000 cases later. *Ann Surg* 208:435-442, 1988.
3. Donaldson MC, Mannick JA, Whittemore AD: Femoral distal bypass with in situ greater saphenous vein: Long-term results using the Mills valvulotome. *Ann Surg* 213:115-121, 1991.
4. Gupta SK, Veith FJ: Inadequacy of diagnosis related group (DRG) reconstructions. *J Vasc Surg* 11:348-357, 1990.
5. Rosenthal D, Dickson C, Rodriguez FJ, et al: Infrainguinal endovascular in situ saphenous vein bypass: Ongoing results. *J Vasc Surg* 20:389-395, 1994.

CHAPTER 10

The Current Role of a Supervised Exercise Program as Therapy for Arterial Claudication

Robert B. Patterson, M.D.
Associate Professor of Surgery, Associate Surgeon-in-Chief; Chief, Peripheral Vascular Surgery; Medical Director, Vascular Exercise Program; Co-director, Noninvasive Vascular Laboratory, Department of Surgery, Division of Vascular Surgery, Brown University School of Medicine, Providence, Rhode Island; The Miriam Hospital, Providence, Rhode Island

Andrea M. Colucci, R.N.
Vascular Nurse Clinician, The Miriam Hospital, Providence, Rhode Island

Christina M. Braun, R.N.
Vascular Nurse Clinician, The Miriam Hospital, Providence, Rhode Island

By the year 2000, 13% of the population will be 65 years of age or older; by 2030, this will increase to 22%.[1] Attendant on this aging is a need to maintain the health and independence of these individuals. Eighty percent of individuals older than age 65 years have one or more chronic illnesses, and half describe lifestyle limitations ranging from minor to severe.[2] Many of the frequent causes for disability (e.g., visual impairment, arthritis, and back pain) are not among the major causes of death. Thus, the physiologic consequences of the aging process limit the enjoyment of life at a stage when many individuals are now expecting to enjoy the freedom of time and maturity to which they have devoted their working lives.

Arterial claudication represents an increasing threat to the mobility and independence of this aging population. Although the natural history of this disease is relatively benign from the standpoint of risk of amputation, the cost in terms of mobility, health perceptions, and associated disease processes is high. The observation that participation in supervised exercise improves the symptoms of claudication in patients without the need for surgical or endovascular intervention has been verified by several investigators.[3-7] Studies of health perceptions and well-being have identified patients with claudication as having self-perceptions of health that are significantly depressed from an age-matched population; responses are equivalent to those from patients with other debilitating diseases such as chronic low back pain and congestive heart failure.[8] Although optimal methods for assessing the quality of life in patients with peripheral arterial disease have not been established, the Short-Form-36 (SF-36) has generally been accepted as a valid survey instrument.[9] Studies using SF-36 responses consistently demonstrate an impairment in quality-of-life measures in patients with intermittent claudication when compared with healthy, age-matched controls.

Invasive interventions have been endorsed by an interdisciplinary committee[10] as therapy for incapacitating claudication, but angioplasty and surgery each carry costs, in terms of both health care dollars and potential morbidity, that do not support their widespread and indiscriminate application. Additionally, interventional therapies applied without attempting to address the associated problems of deconditioning and poor exercise tolerance in patients with claudication will not provide the comprehensive care this population needs. Exercise training has proved to be effective in improving objective treadmill performance[3] and community-based walking ability.[4] In the only well-controlled randomized studies comparing angioplasty vs. exercise as therapy for claudication, at 18-months' follow-up, the group participating in exercise had superior results to those having undergone angioplasties,[11] and at a 6-year follow up, there was no difference in results between the groups.[12]

To expand the potential therapies available to our patients, we instituted a program of supervised vascular exercise in 1993. Research from this program has documented an improvement in treadmill walking ability of greater than 250% and an improvement in the Physical Function subscale, Bodily Pain subscale, and Physical Composite Score as measured by SF-36. More importantly, however, the greatest benefit of our clinical exercise program has been the ability to offer effective alternative therapy for claudication to our patients, allowing us to reserve invasive intervention for those patients who have not achieved adequate improvement with the program.

COMPONENTS OF THE BROWN VASCULAR EXERCISE PROGRAM

The optimal method for training patients with arterial claudication to walk better has not been elucidated. The components that were most important from a meta-analysis of exercise therapy[3] were (1) intermittent exercise to near maximal pain, (2) a program duration of 6 months, and (3) walking as the mode of exercise. Our program design incorporates these factors but is of lesser duration; we have found a program length of 12 weeks is better tolerated and less expensive to administer and provides excellent short and long-term benefits.[6] The program is focused on increasing pain-free walking distance and improving total fitness in an elderly, deconditioned population. The addition of lectures, cardiovascular conditioning, and muscle toning to treadmill training promotes patient and family education, an improvement in the cardiopulmonary reserve, and a decrease in cardiovascular risk.

PERSONNEL AND EQUIPMENT REQUIREMENTS

The program medical director is a board-certified vascular surgeon (RBP) with a long-standing interest in the nonoperative management of patients with arterial claudication. A vascular internist, cardiologist, or geriatrician could also serve as medical director for a program, depending on local interest and practice structure. We currently share a 1.0 full-time equivalent nursing position between two registered nurses (AC and CB) and believe strongly that a nurse is critical to the safe and clinically appropriate maintenance of the program. A background in critical care or cardiac rehabilitation (or both) is ideal, and certification in advanced cardiac life support is an additional benefit. Advanced training and certification in clinical exercise physiology through the American College of Sports Medicine is available and has proven useful in both clinical and research settings.

An exercise physiologist assists us in supervising the exercise sessions and in helping develop individual exercise prescriptions. Undergraduate and masters candidates from the University of Rhode Island Department of Physical Education and Exercise Science have interned with this program, using it as independent study to meet their educational needs. This role could be filled or supplemented by a physical therapist, which potentially would expand the use of personnel and equipment to provide postoperative rehabilitation as well.

SPACE AND RESOURCES

Exercise training takes place in a dedicated 750-sq ft exercise room with four Landice #8700 treadmills (speed, 0.5-11 mph; grade, 0-15 degrees), three Schwinn Air-Dyne bikes, four Schwinn DX 900 bicycle ergometers, two Monarch upper body ergometers, one Combi electronic bicycle ergometer, and free weights for strength training. This is sufficient for eight patients, and the class size is dictated by the number of treadmills. Bicycle stress testing is performed in a dedicated space (60 sq ft) using an electronic Bosch Model ERG 551 bicycle ergometer (work load in Watts) with a stress test monitor (Quinton 3000 ECG and oscilloscope) and is done under the supervision of the cardiology consultant. A Medgraphics metabolic cart is available and is used in collaborative research studies but is not necessary to support the clinical exercise program.

PROGRAM STRUCTURE

The program is divided into three phases: pretesting, training, and maintenance. Although the exercise therapy used in our clinical program is the same as in our research protocols, our criteria for participation are more liberal, that is, no one is automatically excluded because of age or comorbid disease. We receive patient referrals from primary care physicians (i.e., family practitioners and general internists), vascular surgeons, cardiologists, and interventional radiologists, as well as receiving requests from the patients themselves. Pretesting includes a nursing evaluation, a noninvasive lower extremity vascular examination, progressive treadmill testing, and cardiac screening. Before the nursing evaluation, a written referral is required from the patient's primary care physician. This ensures open communication with the primary care physician, who otherwise may be unaware of the patient's referral for therapy if initiated by another specialist or by the patient himself.

PHASE 1
Nursing Evaluation
Because the long-term success of exercise therapy is so closely linked to patient commitment and because the superior results of supervised programs are most likely also due to increased compliance, the role of the supervising nurse is critical to the program's success. A strong professional bond develops between the patients and the nurse director, initiated during the nursing evaluation, when a general medical and surgical history is completed. The date of the onset of symptoms is determined to eliminate patients having symptoms of claudication for less than 3 months, as this population may experience improvement without intervention.[13] The location of the pain, the estimated walking distance, and the time to relief with rest are also documented. This information defines the patients' perceptions of their disease and helps them establish goals and objectives for improvement in activities of daily living. In addition to the measurement of vital signs, a lower

extremity assessment is completed that includes an evaluation of distal pulses, capillary refill rate, and the presence or absence of rubor. Patients with symptoms of ischemic rest pain or physical signs of advanced ischemia such as pallor with elevation and dependent rubor are referred to the program medical director for evaluation before further testing. If limb-threatening ischemia is present, the primary care physician is consulted for further evaluation and follow-up.

Noninvasive Vascular Testing
If the patient meets the clinical criteria as established in the nursing assessment, the results of standard noninvasive vascular testing are reviewed. Patients with resting ankle–brachial ratios of less than 0.9 and decreases in ankle pressure of 15 mm Hg after 5 minutes of treadmill walking are considered eligible for entrance into the program. Patients who do not meet these hemodynamic criteria are referred to the medical director to determine whether there may be another cause to their pain complex (e.g., spinal stenosis or arthritis).

Cardiac Screening
Patients entering the program are required to undergo cardiac screening, which is essential in identifying signs and symptoms of coronary artery disease that may otherwise be silent. This defines the potential cardiac risk associated with varying work loads and assists in establishing the appropriate intensities for exercise prescription. Because standard treadmill testing by the Bruce or modified Bruce protocol is of little value in these patients because of their inability to sustain walking long enough to reach an exercise heart rate, screening includes either bicycle exercise testing or pharmacologic stress testing with myocardial perfusion imaging. Because of patients' increased susceptibility to fatigue and poor strength, increased time is required to reach steady state in this elderly population.[14] Bicycle testing protocols should start at a low intensity and should include a warm-up period, a small rise in work load, and stages consisting of 2 or more minutes each. We have observed that these patients are able to complete 6 or more minutes of exercise on a low-level bicycle-testing protocol. Bicycle stress tests are reviewed by the consulting cardiologist, and patients who are determined ineligible are referred back to their primary care physician for further evaluation.

Progressive Treadmill Test
Progressive treadmill testing is superior to static load treadmill testing in assessing the response to therapy. The most popular

tests[15,16] are difficult for our frail, elderly patients because the starting treadmill speed is 2 mph. We have devised a progressive treadmill test (PTT) of variable speed and grade, the initial stages of which are less demanding (Table 1), and have validated this protocol against the constant speed, progressive load test of Hiatt[16]

TABLE 1.
Progressive Treadmill Test

Minutes	Stage 1	Meters
1		26.8
2	1 mph	53.6
3	5%	80.5
4		107.3
5		134.1
Stage 2		
6		174.3
7		214.6
8	1.5 mph	254.8
9	10%	295.0
10		335.3
Stage 3		
11		388.9
12		442.6
13	2 mph	496.2
14	10%	549.9
15		603.5
Stage 4		
16		670.6
17		737.6
18	2.5 mph	804.7
19	10%	871.7
20		938.8
Stage 5		
21		1005.8
22		1072.9
23	2.5 mph	1140.0
24	15%	1207.0
25		1274.1

(unpublished data). The PTT is performed to obtain objective measurements of distal pressures before and after exercise, to ensure that all patients entering the program meet the hemodynamic inclusion criteria and to determine a starting point for exercise prescription.

Before beginning the PTT, distal pressures are measured and ankle–brachial indices (ABIs) are calculated. The patient begins walking and progresses through each 5-minute stage with increasing intensity. Vital signs are recorded at the end of each stage. The PTT measures the variables of time walked to the onset of symptoms (claudicatory pain time [CPT]) and time walked to limiting claudication (maximum walking time) on a claudicatory pain scale of 0 to 4, where 4 equals maximum tolerable pain. Once at maximum pain, the patient lies supine, and distal pulses are recorded and re-recorded every 2 minutes until hemodynamic recovery time, which reflects the time required for ankle pressure indices to return to baseline measurements. Concurrently, the symptomatic recovery time is documented and reflects the time elapsed to self-perceived pain relief.

PHASE 2
Exercise Sessions

After completion of the pretesting phase, the patient enters phase 2, the 12-week supervised exercise program. Exercise sessions are of 1-hour duration three times a week for 12 weeks. The 1-hour exercise session begins with static stretching of all major muscle groups, which is essential for improving and maintaining flexibility.[17] After group stretches are completed, half of the class begins treadmill training while the others begin cardiovascular training. Each patient's starting work load for treadmill training is determined by the time and intensity walked on the PTT at entry. They begin their treadmill walking at a speed and grade that produces onset of claudication within a 3- to 5-minute period. They are then instructed to walk to near maximum pain, pause the treadmill, and record the time walked. Patients are instructed to remain standing until pain free and to repeat the walk–pause cycle until the 20-minute training period is completed. At the end of the training period, CPT and total time walked during the 20 minutes is evaluated. When patients are able to walk 5 minutes without stopping for two consecutive sessions, the speed or grade is increased, which most patients are able to achieve after 2 weeks of training.

Because the intensity of exercise is systematically increased every 2 weeks, patients perceive that they continue walking less than 5-minute intervals. This apparent lack of progress can be very frustrating. To allow patients to appreciate their progress, after 6 weeks of training, we test patients at the original speed and grade walked at entry. CPT and total walking time are compared to the first session, and most patients able to walk 20 minutes at their original speed and grade without experiencing claudication. After 12 weeks of training, patients are retested at the speed and grade they were walking at midterm, and total walking time is reevaluated. These midterm and final walk tests are completed strictly for individual motivation and are not to be confused with the PTT completed at entry, graduation, and annually.

While half the class is training on the treadmill, the second half of the class is performing cardiovascular exercises, included to improve endurance and cardiopulmonary status. The time and intensity of cardiovascular training is determined by preexisting medical conditions, exercise tolerance, entrance stress test results, and recommendations by our consulting cardiologist. However, our average patient with claudication has been able to begin with 12 minutes of cardiovascular training using stationary biking, Air-Dyne biking, rowing, or arm cycling and has been able to progress to 20 minutes by week 4. At the end of the session, all participants assemble for group muscle toning using light handheld weights and then repeat stretching of all major muscle groups.

This elderly population often has been inactive and deconditioned for an extended period of time. Although improvement in pain-free walking distance is the main goal of the program, we believe that adding cardiovascular training such as biking, rowing, and muscle toning helps improve total fitness and enables patients to better perform activities of daily living.

Education Lectures

In addition to improving physical conditioning, patients attend weekly education lectures that provide information enabling patients to make healthy lifestyle changes and modify risk factors associated with peripheral vascular disease. These lectures address risk factors for atherosclerosis and their modification and include overviews of nutrition, exercise, and potential complications of atherosclerotic cardiovascular disease, specifically covering warning signs and symptoms. Lecture topics include Heart Healthy Eating, Foot Care, Diabetes, Arthritis, Body Mechanics, Benefits of Exercise, and the Natural History of Claudication. Because these patients often experience chronic pain from other conditions compounding the discomfort of their claudication, inclusion of topics such as Management of Arthritis and Body Mechanics helps patients identify and manage associated problems that may interfere with their training.

PHASE 3

The last phase involves maintenance: exercise training as an alternative to surgery is a lifelong commitment, and all graduates are encouraged to continue regular exercise for claudication a minimum of 3 days/week. On completion of the 12-week program, all patients are offered an ongoing, supervised maintenance program providing flexible hours at an affordable rate, allowing them the opportunity to keep in contact with their classmates and enjoy the security of a familiar, experienced staff. Patients who choose not to participate in maintenance at our facility often make arrangements to attend a local health club or YMCA. All patients are followed up annually with repeat PTTs and nursing interviews and are encouraged to call the staff for advice or questions about problems occurring during the intervals between follow-up periods.

RESULTS

PATIENT POPULATION

From May 1993 to January 1999, 117 patients between the ages of 45 and 85 years with symptoms of arterial claudication for greater than 3 months have participated in the Brown Vascular Exercise Program. This reflects a typical population of patients with claudication and co-morbid diseases including controlled diabetes, stable heart disease, arthritis, hypertension, chronic obstructive pulmonary disease (COPD), and chronic renal insufficiency. We have successfully treated patients with end-stage COPD, chronic congestive heart failure, hemodialysis-dependent renal failure, and blindness, although they have been excluded from our research protocols. Obviously, these special populations of patients with claudication require extensive personal attention and modification of their exercise protocols. Although claudication is initially identified as the primary activity limitation of all participants, co-morbid diseases frequently become more limiting as walking tolerance increases. Advice from and collaboration with other physicians involved in exercise training as therapy for congestive heart failure and COPD have been invaluable. The wide range of resting ABIs (0.21-0.95; mean, 0.46) at entrance reflects the lack of relationship between hemodynamics and symptoms,[18-20] and, indeed, the ABI at entry has had no correlation with outcomes in our experience.

WALKING ABILITY

Data from the PTT at entry and on program completion were available for 86 graduates, and results were available from 1- and 2-year follow-up evaluations for 22. The average maximum distance patients were able to walk on entry to the program was 184 m (range, 28-938 m) (Fig 1), primarily representing the distance completed during stage 1 of the PTT. After 12 weeks of training, the average patient walked 580 m, which reflects a threefold improvement over baseline, and walked at stage 3 or greater of the PTT, which is a much higher exercise intensity than that achieved at entry. The average treadmill distance walked for the 22 patients with long-term data available was 251 m at program entry, 772 m on program completion, 882 m at the first year, and 731 m at the 2-year follow-up (Fig 2), which indicates that the majority of patients were able to maintain their threefold improvement over baseline.

In follow-up evaluations of up to 5 years, nine patients have undergone lower extremity intervention—five for claudication (three had angioplasties and two had surgery) and four for limb salvage—and there has been one primary amputation in a patient with diabetes and end-stage renal disease, 5 years after the program's completion. Seven patients have had myocardial infarctions, and eight patients have died (four from cardiac causes, two from cancer, and two from unknown causes).

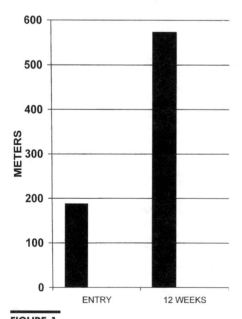

FIGURE 1.
Walking distance at entry and after 12 weeks of supervised exercise therapy (n = 86).

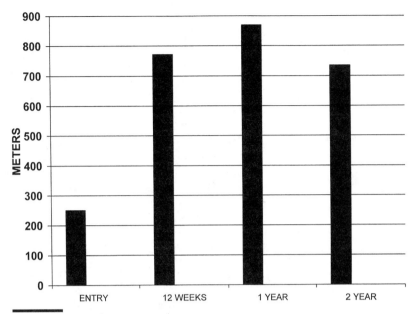

FIGURE 2.
Walking distance with a 2-year follow-up after 12 weeks of supervised exercise therapy (n = 22).

QUALITY-OF-LIFE MEASUREMENTS

In our study comparing home-based exercise (HOMEX) with supervised exercise (SUPEX),[6] there were no differences at baseline between treatment groups on the eight standard subscales of Physical Function, Role-Physical Function, Pain Index, General Health, Vitality Score, Social Function, Role-Emotional, or Mental Health (Table 2). Similarly, composite scores for the physical and mental components and the three individual walking items were no different at baseline.

On completion of the program, the scores on the Physical Function and the Bodily Pain subscales, the composite score on the physical component, and the scores for the three walking items (walking 1+ miles, walking many blocks, and walking 1 block) improved for both the SUPEX and the HOMEX groups ($P < 0.01$), and there were no intergroup differences. This improvement was unchanged at follow-up for both groups (Table 2). The lack of differences between the HOMEX and SUPEX groups in improvement in quality-of-life measures were not surprising given the rigorous nature of our control group. To replicate a clinical program of exercise therapy for claudication and to control solely for the effects of exercise supervision, we exposed the HOMEX group to the same series of weekly lectures as our SUPEX group. The patients' degree

TABLE 2.
Value of a Supervised Exercise Program

	Baseline		Program Completion		6-Month Follow-up	
	SUPEX	HOMEX	SUPEX	HOMEX	SUPEX	HOMEX
Physical Function	43 ± 17.7	41 ± 20.8	52 ± 22.2*	53 ± 24.4*	56 ± 14.4*	54 ± 23.5*
Role-Physical Function	45 ± 42.2	30 ± 34.7	44 ± 42.2	49 ± 41.6	49 ± 39.7	45 ± 41.0
Pain Index	53 ± 20.8	51 ± 20.6	64 ± 23.6*	61 ± 21.6*	62 ± 20.6*	64 ± 19.3*
General Health	64 ± 18.9	60 ± 23.0	65 ± 16.8	62 ± 22.8	64 ± 13.8	64 ± 22.5
Vitality Score	52 ± 19.9	46 ± 18.9	53 ± 16.9	57 ± 15.9	54 ± 17.9	55 ± 19.5
Social Function	81 ± 22.8	80 ± 21.1	87 ± 15.2	82 ± 17.6	81 ± 18.3	88 ± 14.6
Role-Emotional Health	71 ± 36.6	76 ± 33.8	72 ± 36.3	74 ± 33.3	70 ± 36.0	77 ± 32.6
Mental Health	72 ± 18.8	70 ± 18.3	74 ± 14.8	77 ± 13.6	72 ± 16.1	78 ± 13.8
Standard Physical Component	35 ± 7.1	33 ± 9.4	38 ± 8.3*	38 ± 12.0*	39 ± 8.6*	38 ± 11.1*
Standard Mental Component	53 ± 9.6	53 ± 9.0	53 ± 8.3	54 ± 8.2	51 ± 10.2	55 ± 7.3
Walk 1+ Miles	1.2 ± 0.5	1.2 ± 0.5	1.3 ± 0.5*	1.5 ± 0.7*	1.3 ± 0.5*	1.5 ± 0.6*
Walk Many Blocks	1.26 ± 0.5	1.39 ± 0.6	1.75 ± 0.7*	1.96 ± 0.8*	1.72 ± 0.7*	1.75 ± 0.8*
Walk 1 Block	1.70 ± 0.7	1.86 ± 0.7	2.04 ± 0.9*	2.52 ± 0.7*	2.44 ± 0.5*	2.45 ± 0.8*

Note: There was no statistically significant intergroup difference at any interval.
*Difference from baseline, $P < 0.01$.

Abbreviations: HOMEX, home-based exercise; *SUPEX,* supervised exercise.

(Courtesy of Patterson RB, Pinto B, Marcus B, et al: Value of a supervised exercise program for the therapy of arterial claudication. *J Vasc Surg* 25:312-319, 1997. By permission.)

of home exercise was monitored by asking them to maintain weekly activity logs that were reviewed at each lecture session with the program nurse. They also were afforded the opportunity to have individual exercise counseling with the nurse at these sessions to answer questions regarding their activity and progress. Both groups received far more intervention than is customarily available to patients seen by their primary physician or surgeon for symptoms of intermittent claudication.

EXPERIENCE WITH STARTING A PROGRAM

Developing a vascular exercise program often proves to be a challenge. Retaining administrative support, financing, and reimbursement are difficult issues to resolve in these fiscally challenging times. Sharing expenses with another program can greatly defray costs by using equipment and personnel in a more efficient fashion. Although cardiac rehabilitation programs are the most obvious affiliation, we have found that the very different exercise protocols, philosophies, and training of cardiac rehabilitation nurses and physicians often are at odds with vascular exercise and may prove to be a barrier early in the development of the program. We chose to affiliate with an existing weight management program, and this allowed us to preserve our own identity, maintain adequate class time, and defray costs. Affiliation with physical therapy programs has also been successful. When consolidating with another program, it is important to be aware of the treadmill specifications necessary for training patients with claudication. Treadmills used for vascular exercise must begin at a speed of 0.5 mph, increase in increments of 0.1 mph, have an elevation control, and have a pause feature that must be at least 10 minutes in length to accommodate the various recovery periods between training intervals in patients with claudication.

REIMBURSEMENT

Obtaining third-party reimbursement is a somewhat onerous task, predominately because, as a discrete therapy, exercise therapy for claudication does not yet have a separate Current Procedural Terminology code and is therefore not nationally recognized as a defined therapy. The majority of our patients qualify for partial coverage of individual program components, which includes reimbursement for pretesting such as the PTT, noninvasive vascular testing, and cardiac screening. This leaves the average patient with an affordable out-of-pocket expense for the 36 exercise sessions. More importantly, because the success and economic efficiency of our program is recognized by local third-party insurers, we have obtained full coverage by a local HMO as a test case and are negotiating with other payers based on the data we have accrued. Strategies to increase reimbursement that have proven successful for other programs (personal communications) include supervision and billing through physical therapy, providing "health club" services and membership structure, and supplementing program income through "elderly fitness" programs. Initial funding from intramural and extramural grants for research on claudication permitted the start-up costs of our program to be defrayed and allowed us to provide further data to support the efficacy of supervised exercise.[6,21]

DISCUSSION
NATURAL HISTORY
Although the absence of hemodynamic data has brought many older studies of the natural history of claudication into question, Cronenwett et al.[20] followed up 91 male veterans with mild claudication (ABI, 0.40-0.91; mean, 0.63) for 2.5 years and reported 12% with symptom improvement, 28% with unchanged symptoms, and 60% with worsening symptoms. Twenty patients underwent surgery (7 for claudication and 13 for limb salvage), which yielded an annual intervention rate of 9%. Ten patients died (7 from cardiac causes, 2 from cancer, and 1 from unknown causes), which yielded an annual mortality of 4.8%. McAllister,[22] in 1976, reported a retrospective review of patients with claudication and occlusive disease confirmed by arteriography. At an average of 6 years of follow-up, 52% were improved and 26% were stable. The excessive incidence of co-morbid vascular conditions, many with more profound potential effects on the quality of life, is evident from long-term follow-up data from the Framingham study by Kannel.[23] Within 10 years of the onset of claudicatory symptoms, 60% of patients had died. Of those free of disease at the onset of claudicatory symptoms, 43% subsequently had coronary heart disease, 24% subsequently had heart failure, and 21% subsequently had strokes.

DRUG THERAPY
An effective drug regimen for the treatment of claudication remains the Holy Grail of vascular internists, cardiologists, and pharmaceutical companies. The promise of an oral agent to improve the symptoms of claudication has not been realized, despite numerous studies and much research. Early investigations of vasodilators (e.g., tolazoline, nylidrin, and isoxsuprine) suggested that they were ineffective as therapy for claudication.[24] Pentoxifylline is frequently prescribed, and meta-analyses of the available literature[5,25] suggest a statistically significant objective

improvement in the distance walked by patients with claudication receiving pentoxifylline compared with placebo. The additive role of pentoxifylline to exercise[26] failed to demonstrate a benefit at program completion (exercise improvement, 178%; exercise plus pentoxifylline, 204%). Unfortunately, the expense, incidence of gastrointestinal side effects, and limited clinical effectiveness[27-29] has led to a diminished enthusiasm for its use.

The recent introduction of cilostazol, an inhibitor of type II phosphodiesterase activity in platelets and with adjunctive vasodilatory properties, has regenerated interest in the pharmacologic therapies. Results from a multicenter trial[30] of cilostazol vs. placebo are strikingly similar to those of pentoxifylline: there is a statistically significant improvement in walking distance that is of undetermined clinical efficacy. In fact, reviewing all the drug trials for claudication suggests that, given the strong positive effect seen in many studies, placebo may be the most cost-effective pharmacotherapy, albeit one with an unacceptable incidence of untoward side effects.

EXERCISE THERAPY

Many novel therapies for arterial claudication have fallen from favor: Achilles' tendon sectioning, lumbar sympathectomy, selective crushing of the peripheral nerves to the calf muscles, heel lifts, and subcutaneous implantation of amniotic membranes.[31] The role of exercise, however, has been recognized as effective since the 1960s,[7,32] although the structure of an exercise program and its components vary greatly.[3] Other's experience with supervised exercise[33] mirrors our own, supporting the importance of supervision over home-based therapy or simple office instructions. The possible mechanisms of action that contribute to the success of exercise remain elusive and have been nicely reviewed by Regensteiner et al.[33] These include improvement in local blood flow through changes in viscosity, redistribution of flow, improved oxidative metabolism of skeletal muscles, and changes in gait with exercise training.

Concerns about the adverse effects of exercise training, especially with respect to the effects of repetitive exercise on claudicatory pain, have been raised by some authors. These include exacerbation of the chronic denervation seen in peripheral arterial disease,[34] but a subsequent report by the same group[35] found progression of peripheral neuropathy in patients with occlusive disease that was unaffected by participation in supervised exercise. Others have suggested that the repetitive ischemia–reperfusion injuries caused by intermittent claudication may incite an inflammatory response that could accelerate atherosclerosis. Tisi and his colleagues[36,37] have confirmed that inflammatory markers (e.g., C-reactive protein, serum amyloid A protein, and the urinary albumin–creatinine ratio) were elevated in patients with claudication compared with a control population but were decreased in a cohort of patients with claudication randomly assigned to exercise.

The benefits of percutaneous transluminal angioplasty and endovascular revascularization in terms of improving claudicatory symptoms and quality of life have been called into question[38,39] because intermediate and late results of intervention are prospectively obtained with functional assessment tools. In the only randomized study of exercise therapy vs. angioplasty with long-term

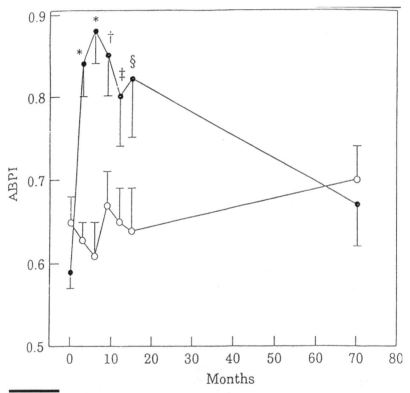

FIGURE 3.
Median (ABPI) vs. time in patients randomly assigned to percutaneous transluminal angioplasty (*closed circle*) or exercise therapy (*open circle*) (standard error bars) $^*P$ = 0.0001, $^\dagger P$ = 0.001, $^\ddagger P$ = 0.05, $^\S P$ = 0.02 (Wilcoxon paired test). (Reprinted from Perkins JM, Collin J, Creasy TS, et al: Exercise training versus angioplasty for stable claudication. Long and medium term results of a prospective, randomised trial. *Eur J Vasc Endovasc Surg* 11():409-413, copyright 1996, by permission of the publisher W B Saunders Company Limited London.)

follow-up,[12] an early improvement in ABIs was noted in the angio-plasty group (Fig 3). This did not correlate with improvement in walking ability, which was far greater in the exercise group at intermediate follow-up (Fig 4). Disappointingly, however, at late follow-up (70 months), the improvements in ABIs and walking ability had been lost, and very few of the patients were exercising with any regularity. Clearly, more controlled trials with greater numbers are required to establish the relative value of exercise and angioplasty in the overall management of intermittent claudica-tion, as well as to identify subgroups that should preferentially be offered either therapy.[38,40]

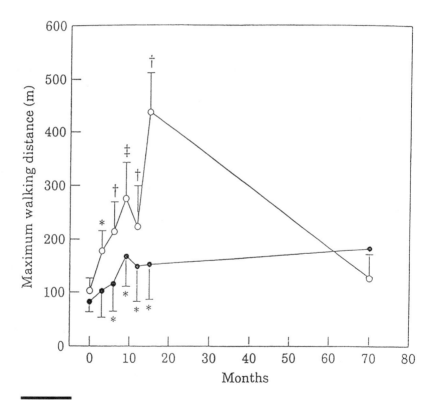

FIGURE 4.
Median maximum walking distance vs. time in patients randomly assigned to percutaneous transluminal angioplasty (*closed circle*) or exer-cise therapy (*open circle*) (standard error bars). *$P < 0.005$, †$P < 0.001$, ‡$P = 0.0001$ (Wilcoxon paired test). (Reprinted from Perkins JM, Collin J, Creasy TS, et al: Exercise training versus angioplasty for stable claudica-tion. Long and medium term results of a prospective, randomised trial. *Eur J Vasc Endovasc Surg* 11():409-413, copyright 1996, by permission of the publisher W B Saunders Company Limited London.)

CONCLUSION

We consider our program to be optimal in its approach to the treatment of arterial claudication. Five years' experience in training patients with claudication leads us to believe that focusing on the total patient offers the best results in both improved walking distance and the overall state of well-being. Including both psychosocial and clinical components allows a more holistic approach to this patient population. An objective measurement of improved maximum walking distance is convincing, but it is the patients' subjective perception of their progress that has been most remarkable. For example, the average patient with claudication who was initially unable to play golf on retirement is now walking 18 holes without too much difficulty. Elderly patients who had increasingly limited their activities are shopping with friends and visiting family. Interestingly, patients are very satisfied with their improvement in walking, but family members are more impressed by the positive changes in their general health and psychosocial behavior. By including both clinical and psychosocial measures, we are able to stabilize and improve symptoms of claudication, decrease cardiovascular risk, and provide education to patients and family.

REFERENCES

1. Healthy People 2000. (PHS)91-502 12:23-24, 1991.
2. Stemmer EA: Introduction, in Aronow WS, Stemmer EA, Wilson SE (eds): *Vascular Disease in the Elderly.* Armonk, NY, Futura Publishing, 1997, pp 1-10.
3. Gardner AW, Poehlman ET: Exercise rehabilitation programs for the treatment of claudication pain: A meta-analysis. *JAMA* 274:975-980, 1995.
4. Hiatt WR, Regensteiner JG, Hargarten ME, et al: Benefit of exercise conditioning for patients with peripheral arterial disease. *Circulation* 81:602-609, 1990.
5. McDaniel MD: A 52-year-old woman with diabetes and claudication (clinical conference). *JAMA* 279:615-621, 1998.
6. Patterson RB, Pinto B, Marcus B, et al: Value of a supervised exercise program for the therapy of arterial claudication. *J Vasc Surg* 25:312-319, 1997.
7. Skinner JS, Strandness DE: Exercise and intermittent claudication: Effect of physical training. *Circulation* 36:23-29, 1967.
8. Murphy TP: Medical outcomes studies in peripheral vascular disease. *J Vasc Interv Radiol* 9:879-889, 1998.
9. Stewart AL, Greenfield S, Hays RD, et al: Functional status and well-being of patients with chronic conditions: Results from the medical outcomes study. *JAMA* 262:907-913, 1989.
10. Pentecost MJ, Criqui MH, Dorros G, et al: Guidelines for peripheral percutaneous transluminal angioplasty of the abdominal aorta and lower extremity vessels. *Circulation* 89:511-531, 1994.

11. Creasy TS, McMillan PJ, Fletcher EW, et al: Is percutaneous transluminal angioplasty better than exercise for claudication? Preliminary results from a prospective randomised trial. *Eur J Vasc Surg* 4:135-140, 1990.

12. Perkins JM, Collin J, Creasy TS, et al: Exercise training versus angioplasty for stable claudication. Long and medium term results of a prospective, randomised trial. *Eur J Vasc Endovasc Surg* 11:409-413, 1996.

13. Imparato A: Perspective: Intermittent claudication. *J Vasc Surg* 2:767-768, 1985.

14. Skinner JS: Importance of aging for exercise testing and exercise prescription, in Skinner J (ed): *Exercise Testing and Exercise Prescription for Special Cases*. Philadelphia, Lea and Febinger, 1987, pp 67-75.

15. Gardner AW, Skinner JS, Cantwell BW, et al: Progressive vs. single-stage treadmill tests for evaluation of claudication. *Med Sci Sports Exerc* 23:402-408, 1991.

16. Hiatt WR, Nawaz D, Regensteiner JG, et al: The evaluation of exercise performance in patients with peripheral vascular disease. *J Cardiopulm Rehabil* 12:525-532, 1988.

17. Durnstine LJ, King AC, Painter PL, et al: Flexibility/range of motion, in American College of Sports Medicine (ed): *Resource Guidelines for Exercise Testing and Prescription*. Philadelphia, Lea and Febiger, 1993, pp 327-336.

18. Bowers BL, Valentine RJ, Myers SI, et al: The natural history of patients with claudication with toe pressures of 40 mm Hg or less. *J Vasc Surg* 18:506-511, 1993.

19. Fowl RJ, Gewirtz RJ, Love MC, et al: Natural history of claudicants with critical hemodynamic indices. *Ann Vasc Surg* 6:31-33, 1992.

20. Cronenwett JL, Warner KG, Zelenock GB, et al: Intermittent claudication: Current results of nonoperative management. *Arch Surg* 119:430-436, 1984.

21. Pinto B, Marcus B, Patterson RB, et al: On-site versus home exercise programs: Psychological benefits for individuals with arterial claudication. *J Aging Phys Activity* October:311-328, 1997.

22. McAllister FF: The fate of patients with intermittent claudication managed nonoperatively. *Am J Surg* 132:593-595, 1976.

23. Kannel WB: The demographics of claudication and the aging of the American population. *Vasc Med* 1:60-64, 1996.

24. Coffman JD, Mannick JA: Failure of vasodilator drugs in arteriosclerosis obliterans. *Ann Intern Med* 76:35-39, 1972.

25. Girolami B, Bernardi E, Prins MH, et al: Treatment of intermittent claudication with physical training, smoking cessation, pentoxifylline, or nafronyl: A meta-analysis. *Arch Intern Med* 159:337-345, 1999.

26. Ernst E, Kollar L, Reach KL: Does pentoxifylline prolong the walking distance in exercise claudicants? A placebo-controlled double-blind trial. *Angiology* 43:121-125, 1992.

27. Hood SC, Moher D, Barber GG: Management of intermittent claudication with pentoxifylline: Meta-analysis of randomized controlled trials. *CMAJ* 155:1053-1059, 1996.

28. Johnson G Jr: Pentoxifylline and claudication. *J Vasc Surg* 8:649, 1988.
29. Green RM, McNamara J: The effects of pentoxifylline on patients with intermittent claudication. *J Vasc Surg* 7:356-362, 1988.
30. Money SR, Herd JA, Isaacsohn JL, et al: Effect of cilostazol on walking distances in patients with intermittent claudication caused by peripheral vascular disease. *J Vasc Surg* 27:267-275, 1998.
31. Anonymous: Intermittent claudication (editorial). *BMJ* 1:1165-1166, 1976.
32. Larsen DA, Lassen NA: Effects of daily muscular exercise in patients with intermittent claudication. *Lancet* 2:1093-1096, 1966.
33. Regensteiner JG, Meyer TJ, Krupski WC, et al: Hospital vs. home-based exercise rehabilitation for patients with peripheral arterial occlusive disease. *Angiology* 48:291-300, 1997.
34. Regensteiner JG, Wolfel EE, Brass EP, et al: Chronic changes in skeletal muscle histology and function in peripheral arterial disease. *Circulation* 87:413-421, 1993.
35. England JD, Fergusen MA, Hiatt WR, et al: Progression of neuropathy in peripheral vascular disease. *Muscle Nerve* 18:380-387, 1995.
36. Tisi PV, Hulse M, Chulakadabba A, et al: Exercise training for intermittent claudication: Does it adversely affect biochemical markers of the exercise-induced inflammatory response? *Eur J Vasc Endovasc Surg* 14:344-350, 1997.
37. Tisi PV, Shearman CP: The evidence for exercise-induced inflammation in intermittent claudication: Should we encourage patients to stop walking?. *Eur J Vasc Endovasc Surg* 15:7-17, 1998.
38. Whyman MR, Ruckley CV: Should claudicants receive angioplasty or just exercise training? *Cardiovasc Surg* 6:226-231, 1998.
39. Cook TA, Galland RB: Quality of life changes after angioplasty for claudication: Medium-term results affected by comorbid conditions. *Cardiovasc Surg* 5:424-426, 1997.
40. Price JF, Leng GC, Fowkes FG: Should claudicants receive angioplasty or exercise training? *Cardiovasc Surg* 5:463-470, 1997.

PART IV
Anticoagulation

CHAPTER 11

Anticoagulation for Infrainguinal Revascularization

Timur P. Sarac, M.D.
Vascular Surgery Fellow, University of Florida College of Medicine, Division of Vascular Surgery, Gainesville, Florida

James M. Seeger, M.D.
Professor and Chief of Vascular Surgery, University of Florida College of Medicine, Division of Vascular Surgery, Gainesville, Florida

The patency of bypass grafts for infrainguinal revascularization has improved dramatically since Kunlin[1] reported the first lower extremity revascularization using a saphenous vein in 1949. Five-year patency rates of uncomplicated femoropopliteal and infrageniculate bypasses using venous grafts have been reported to be as high as 85%.[2] In contrast, long-term patency rates of infrainguinal bypasses using prosthetic grafts, particularly popliteal and infrageniculate bypasses, are significantly lower; thus, a venous conduit should be used, if at all possible, when such bypasses are required.[3] The reasons for improved patency rates of infrainguinal bypass grafts are multifactorial and include refined technical skills, better selection of patients, and aggressive duplex ultrasound surveillance[4] and pharmacologic measures.[5]

Unfortunately, not all patients undergoing infrainguinal bypasses achieve these good results, and select patients are at significantly increased risk for graft failure. These patients include those with a previous bypass graft failure,[6] those who require bypass grafts constructed from alternative venous conduits because their saphenous veins are inadequate or have been used for other procedures,[7] and those with advanced arterial occlusive disease evidenced by poor distal arterial runoff.[8] Furthermore, graft failure remains a dilemma even for patients without these problems because graft occlusion usually necessitates graft revision, a secondary bypass procedure, or even an amputation.

Although the cause of graft failure (e.g., technical error, intimal hyperplasia, or progressive atherosclerosis) varies with the length of time after the bypass construction, the final common pathway for graft failure is graft thrombosis. Because of this, the use of antithrombotic measures to potentially improve graft patency rates has been explored. This article will review the different antithrombotic measures available to augment patency of lower extremity bypass grafts, with an emphasis on the risk vs. the benefits of each modality. In addition, anticoagulation in the immediate postoperative period and the period after hospital discharge will be discussed separately, as the techniques and risks associated with anticoagulation and the factors associated with bypass graft thrombosis vary significantly between these two time periods.

USE OF ANTICOAGULATION TO IMPROVE EARLY BYPASS GRAFT PATENCY

The patency of arterial bypass grafts is maintained by a balance between the surface thrombogenicity of the bypass graft and the degree of activation of the clotting system in an individual patient. The rate of blood flow through the bypass graft significantly influences this balance by clearing and diluting activated clotting factors from the microenvironment at the graft surface–blood interface, thereby inhibiting progressive thrombus formation. Graft surface thrombogenicity is high immediately after the bypass graft construction, even when a venous conduit is used, and early (within 30 days of bypass construction) bypass graft failure is most often attributed to technical errors that disturb or limit bypass graft flow. Fortunately, the incidence of early bypass graft occlusion in most modern reports is less than 5%. However, in certain circumstances, such as when there is use of marginal venous or prosthetic bypass conduits[3,7] or when there are diseased runoff beds[8] or hypercoagulable states,[9] lower extremity bypass grafts are at increased risk for early failure despite the technical perfection of the bypass procedure.

Antiplatelet agents such as aspirin and dipyridamole have been shown to significantly improve the patency of prosthetic (but not venous) bypass grafts when given preoperatively, and much of the improvement in graft patency rates is due to a decrease in early graft failure (Table 1).[10] Antiplatelet therapy with aspirin also potentially reduces the long-term risk of myocardial infarction and strokes; thus, patients with peripheral arterial occlusive disease

TABLE 1.

Perioperative Anticoagulation Summary

Author	Anticoagulant	Patency
Clyne	Aspirin plus dipyridamole	85% 1-month patency of prosthetic grafts
Becquemin	Ticlopidine	97% 1-week patency of vein grafts
Rutherford	Dextran	93% 1-week patency of high-risk grafts
Sarac	Heparin plus aspirin	97% 1-week patency of high-risk vein grafts
McMillan	LMW heparin	96% 1-week patency of e-PTFE grafts

Abbreviations: LMW, low molecular weight; e-PTFE, expanded polytetrafluoroethylene.

likely benefit from aspirin therapy apart from its effect on early bypass graft patency. In contrast, ticlopidine has been shown to improve vein bypass graft patency, and the difference in patency rates for treated and control grafts continues to increase over time.[11] Nevertheless, antiplatelet agents are not without risks: aspirin administration has been shown to be associated with gastrointestinal and intracranial bleeding, and use of ticlopidine has been associated with diarrhea and, occasionally, hepatotoxic effects.

Low-molecular weight dextran, which acts by inhibiting the factor VIII–von Willebrand factor complex and therefore platelet aggregation, has also been demonstrated to improve early bypass graft patency rates. Rutherford et al.[12] reported that, in patients undergoing lower extremity bypasses potentially at high risk for failure, use of dextran 40 improved 1 week postoperative graft patency rates from 79% to 93% (Table 1). However, by 1 month, patency rates were not different between treated patients and controls. Furthermore, dextran is a volume expander that increases the risk of congestive heart failure, has been reported to cause anaphylactic shock, and can be associated with bleeding complications.

Heparin is also frequently used to attempt to maintain graft patency in the early postoperative period. Apart from their known antithrombin effect of the potentiation of antithrombin III activity, heparin and low-molecular weight heparin have also been demonstrated experimentally to inhibit platelet function.[13] We have recently demonstrated that unfractionated heparin (15 U/kg, continuous infusion to maintain an activated partial thromboplastin time [aPTT] of 1.5 times the control value) begun 6 to 24 hours after an infrainguinal arterial bypass procedure significantly improves early (7-day) graft patency rates (97.3% vs. 85.2%) and limb salvage rates (100% vs. 88.9%) in a subset of patients deemed at high risk for graft failure.[14] The incidence of postoperative wound hematomas in the patients receiving IV heparin in this study was high (32%), but the incidence of wound infection or other wound complications was not increased. Furthermore, almost two thirds of the patients in whom wound hematomas developed had at least one aPTT greater than 106 seconds in the first 48 hours after completion of the bypass procedure.

Low-molecular weight heparin has been shown to potentially improve initial (10-day) bypass graft patency rates compared with unfractionated heparin, although the graft thrombosis rate in the control group that received unfractionated heparin was inordinately high (22%).[15] Low-molecular weight heparin may also reduce the risk of postoperative wound hematomas because of its consistent dose response and may limit intimal hyperplasia because of its smooth muscle antiproliferative effect, although these potential benefits remain to be documented. Regardless, use of low-molecular weight heparin to improve early bypass graft patency is simpler, is not associated with an increased risk of complications compared with IV unfractionated heparin, and can lead to a significant decrease in the hospital stay if long-term anticoagulation is planned.[15]

OUR CURRENT APPROACH TO ANTICOAGULATION IN THE IMMEDIATE POSTOPERATIVE PERIOD

We currently begin 325 mg/day of aspirin preoperatively in all patients undergoing arterial bypass surgery and continue it indefinitely. Furthermore, because of the previously observed high risk of wound hematomas associated with standard dosages of IV unfractionated heparin, we use lower dosages of unfractionated heparin (400-500 U/hr, which results in an aPTT of 1.25 times control values or less) during the first 24 hours of the postoperative period. Subsequently, the heparin dosage is increased by increments of 200 to 300 U/hr until an aPTT of 1.5 times the control value is achieved by 48 to 72 hours after surgery. Heparin boluses are avoided if at all possible. Whether this approach will reduce the risk of postoperative wound hematomas while maintaining the improvement in early graft patency seen with standard-dose unfractionated heparin therapy remains to be determined. However, a randomized trial of standard-dose unfractionated heparin, low-dose unfractionated heparin, and low-molecular weight heparin used in the early postoperative period in patients at high risk for graft failure is currently under way.

USE OF ANTICOAGULATION TO IMPROVE LONG-TERM BYPASS GRAFT PATENCY

Long-term infrainguinal bypass graft failure is also most commonly due to bypass graft thrombosis. Stenosis of the vein bypass graft or graft artery anastomosis due to neointimal hyperplasia or progression of atherosclerotic occlusive disease in the graft inflow or runoff arteries limit and disturb blood flow through the graft, which leads to graft thrombosis. Unfortunately, once bypass graft thrombosis occurs, secondary graft patency is poor despite restoration of graft patency using thrombolysis or thrombectomy and repair of the vein graft or arterial lesion.[16] Because of this, graft replacement is usually required. Duplex ultrasound surveillance of infrainguinal vein bypass grafts has been shown to improve infrainguinal bypass graft patency by allowing detection and repair of graft or arterial stenoses before graft thrombosis; however, this approach is expensive, and graft thrombosis can still occur between surveillance intervals. In addition, no clinically effective method of limiting or eliminating vein graft or anastomotic neointimal hyperplasia exists, and the effect of risk factor modification (e.g., smoking cessation and treatment of hypercholesterolemia) on the progression rate of atherosclerotic arterial occlusive disease remains to be documented.

As previously noted, aspirin has not been shown to improve long-term infrainguinal vein bypass graft patency, and the effect of aspirin therapy on infrainguinal prosthetic bypass graft patency is primarily due to a modest decrease in early graft failure.[10,17] In contrast, Becquemin[11] demonstrated that ticlopidine, an inhibitor of platelet aggregation, improved the 2-year primary and secondary patency rates of femoropopliteal or femorotibial saphenous vein bypass grafts compared with a placebo (secondary patency, 81% vs. 57%) (Table 2). However, there were a significantly greater number of nonischemic adverse events in the patients receiving ticlopidine (primarily diarrhea), and patients taking ticlopidine for prophylaxis against thrombosis after coronary artery stent placement have been found to have increased incidences of bleeding, hepatotoxic effects, and aplastic anemia.[18] Clopidogrel, an

TABLE 2.
Long-term Postoperative Anticoagulation Summary

Author	Anticoagulant	Patency
Antiplatelet Trialists	Aspirin	43% reduction in graft occlusion
Becquemin	Ticlopidine	69% 2-year patency of vein grafts
Kretschmer	Warfarin	80% 5-year patency of femoropopliteal vein grafts
Sarac	Warfarin plus aspirin	81% 3-year patency of vein grafts at high risk for failure

antiplatelet agent similar to ticlopidine, may produce the same improvements in graft patency without the frequency of adverse side effects, but this remains to be documented.[19]

For patients undergoing arterial bypass procedures, long-term anticoagulation with warfarin, which acts by inhibiting vitamin K epoxide reductase, has also been extensively studied. In a recent retrospective study, Seeger et al.[8] found anticoagulation with warfarin to be a predictor of limb salvage in patients undergoing infrainguinal vein bypasses for tissue loss,[8] whereas Harward et al.,[20] in another study from our group, demonstrated anticoagulation with warfarin to improve the long-term patency of infrainguinal arm-vein bypass grafts in patients with critical lower extremity ischemia. Similarly, Flinn et al.[21] have reported that warfarin prolongs the patency of prosthetic infrageniculate bypasses, and, in fact, such bypasses appear to be of clinical value only when long-term anticoagulation with warfarin is used.

In a randomized, prospective trial of patients undergoing femoropopliteal vein bypass grafting, Kretschmer et al.[22] demonstrated improved 5-year secondary patency rates from 57% to 80% and improved 5-year limb salvage rates from 71% to 96% in patients receiving dicumarol. In contrast, in a similar randomized trial, Arfvidsson et al. found that long-term use of dicumarol provided no benefit after infrainguinal vein or prosthetic bypass grafting and was associated with a 5% incidence rate of serious hemorrhagic complications. Johnson et al.[24] also recently found no difference in 4-year primary assisted patency rates of infrainguinal vein bypasses in patients randomly assigned to long-term anticoagulation with warfarin as compared with controls (81% vs. 81%) and also observed an increased number of drug-related complications and an increased mortality rate in the patients randomly assigned to receive warfarin. However, 75% of the patients in Johnson's study who were randomly assigned to the warfarin group either stopped taking the medication or had subtherapeutic international normalized ration (INR) values.[25]

In part, this variability in outcome is likely caused by differences in the risk of graft failure in the patients entered into these trials. If long-term anticoagulation is of value after infrainguinal vein bypass grafting, it should be most beneficial for the subset of patients who are at high risk for bypass graft occlusion. Alternatively, many patients likely do not need adjunctive measures to enhance long-term bypass graft patency, and it does not seem prudent to use long-term anticoagulation in all patients undergoing infrainguinal vein bypass graft procedures given the potential risks of hemorrhagic complications.[26] In the previously described study of perioperative and long-term anticoagulation in

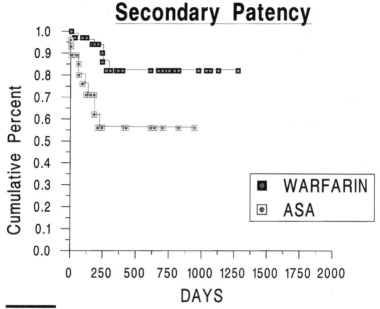

FIGURE 1.
Secondary patency rates by Kaplan-Meier analysis of infrainguinal vein bypass grafts at high risk for failure. Those patients who received warfarin plus aspirin (warfarin) had significantly improved patency rates compared with those who received aspirin (ASA) alone. (Courtesy of Sarac TP, Huber TS, Back MR, et al: Warfarin improves the outcome of infrainguinal vein bypass grafting at high risk for failure. *J Vasc Surg* 28:446-457, 1998. By permission.)

patients at high risk for bypass graft failure from our institution, cumulative 3-year primary, primary assisted, and secondary graft patency rates in patients randomly assigned to warfarin plus aspirin were improved compared with those receiving aspirin alone (Fig 1). Limb salvage rates at 3 years were also improved in the patients who received warfarin plus aspirin (Fig 2). The improved primary assisted and secondary bypass graft patency rates appeared to be caused, in part, by the detection of a significantly greater number of failing grafts as opposed to occluded grafts in the warfarin group compared with the aspirin group. The improvement in the bypass graft patency rate in the patients receiving warfarin plus aspirin was also seen primarily in the first year of follow-up, whereas the improvement in the limb salvage rate continued throughout the 3 years of follow-up (Figs 1 and 2).[14] Potentially, this second observation was due to protection of diseased runoff beds from thrombosis, but this cannot be confirmed. Furthermore, despite a reported risk of long-term hemorrhagic

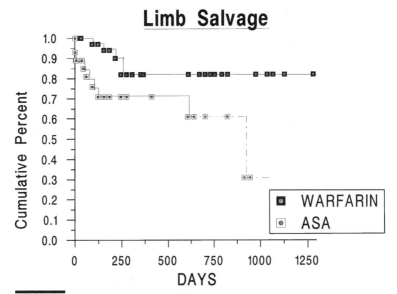

FIGURE 2.
Limb salvage rates by Kaplan-Meier analysis of infrainguinal vein bypass grafts at high risk for failure. Those patients who received warfarin plus aspirin had significantly improved limb salvage compared with those who received aspirin (ASA) alone. (Courtesy of Sarac TP, Huber TS, Back MR, et al: Warfarin improves the outcome of infrainguinal vein bypass grafting at high risk for failure. *J Vasc Surg* 28:446-457, 1998. By permission.)

complications of 7.9 per 100 person-years in patients receiving anticoagulation for stroke prophylaxis,[26] the long-term hemorrhagic complication rates in our study were equivalent between the patients receiving warfarin plus aspirin and those receiving aspirin alone.

OUR CURRENT APPROACH TO LONG-TERM ANTICOAGULATION AFTER AN INFRAINGUINAL BYPASS

Patients with known hypercoagulable states, those deemed at high risk for long-term infrainguinal vein bypass graft failure, and those undergoing infrageniculate bypasses who have minimal remaining venous conduits after the procedure such that graft failure would almost certainly lead to limb loss are currently considered for long-term anticoagulation with warfarin plus aspirin. Patients deemed at high risk for venous bypass graft failures, as previously described, include those with a previous bypass graft failure, those with inadequate saphenous veins, and those with poor distal runoff due to severe distal arterial occlusive disease (Table 3). Patients with a known bleeding diathesis and those at risk for

TABLE 3.
Reasons Why Patients May Have Lower Extremity Bypass Grafts at High
Risk for Failure and/or Limb Loss

1. Hypercoagulable diathesis
2. Diseased runoff bed
3. Poor venous conduit
4. Revision of previously failed bypass graft
5. Prosthetic conduit
6. Tissue loss and minimal remaining venous conduit

intracranial bleeding, such as patients at significant risk for falls, are excluded. Patients at increased risk for hemorrhagic complications, such as those with peptic ulcer disease, are considered for anticoagulation on an individual basis, that is, the risk of bleeding is balanced against the risk of graft failure and subsequent limb loss. Patients undergoing below-knee popliteal or infrageniculate bypasses using prosthetic grafts also undergo long-term anticoagulation with warfarin and aspirin, but very few such bypasses (none in the last several years) are done in our practice. The combined use of warfarin and aspirin is based on the finding that warfarin plus aspirin is more effective in preventing long-term prosthetic heart valve thromboembolic complications as compared with warfarin alone, without increasing the risk of bleeding complications.

Patients selected for long-term anticoagulation are started on aspirin therapy before their bypass procedure, and the aspirin is continued throughout the postoperative period. Most of the patients selected for long-term anticoagulation are also given anticoagulant therapy with heparin in the early postoperative period (as already described). Warfarin administration is begun immediately after the patient resumes intake orally, and heparin anticoagulation is maintained until the INR level is greater than 1.5 to 2.0 (3.0 if the patient has a known hypercoagulable condition). INR values are maintained between 2.0 and 3.0 after hospital discharge for patients without a hypercoagulable condition and are evaluated weekly in our anticoagulant therapy clinics. Once the INR values are stable, biweekly or monthly monitoring is done as long as the INR value remains in the therapeutic range. All patients undergoing infrainguinal bypass procedures (regardless of whether they are receiving long-term anticoagulation) are seen in the outpatient clinic after discharge at 2 weeks, 1 month, 3 months, 6 months, and every 6 months thereafter. Ankle brachial indices and a duplex ultrasound graft scan are obtained before hospital discharge and at all outpatient clinic visits after the initial visit.

Patients found to have failing bypass grafts have their therapy converted back to IV heparin anticoagulation subsequent to arteriography and/or vein graft repair and then again receive warfarin and aspirin for long-term anticoagulation before hospital discharge.

CONCLUSION

Perioperative and long-term anticoagulation appear to be of significant value in select patients undergoing infrainguinal bypass procedures. Patients who benefit from anticoagulation after infrainguinal vein bypasses include those who have a previous infrainguinal bypass that has failed, those without an adequate saphenous vein for use as the bypass conduit, those with poor runoff distal to the bypass, and those with tissue loss in whom all the available venous conduit is being used for the present infrainguinal bypass procedure. Perioperative anticoagulation with IV unfractionated heparin improves early bypass graft patency in such patients. However, it is associated with an increased risk of wound hematomas but not wound infection, and the precise perioperative anticoagulation regimen associated with the least risk of this problem remains undetermined. In contrast, long-term anticoagulation with warfarin and aspirin has been surprisingly safe and appears to be associated with benefits beyond preserving bypass graft patency. Clearly, the final event in infrainguinal bypass graft failure and in progression of arterial occlusive disease is thrombosis, and decreasing the risk of thrombosis in patients, such as those described above with severe peripheral arterial occlusive disease, appears to be warranted.

REFERENCES

1. Kunlin JL: Le traitment de l'arterite obliterante par le greffe veineuse. *Arch Mal Coeur Vaiss* 42:371-374, 1949.
2. Taylor LM, Edwards JM, Porter JM: Present status of reverse vein bypass grafting: Five year results of a modern series. *J Vasc Surg* 11:193-206, 1990.
3. Veith FG, Gupta SK, Ascer E, et al: Six year prospective multicenter randomized comparison of autologous saphenous vein and expanded polytetrafluoroethylene grafts in infrainguinal arterial reconstructions. *J Vasc Surg* 3:104-114, 1986.
4. Mills JL, Bandyk DF, Gahtan V, et al: The origin of infrainguinal vein graft stenosis: A prospective study based on duplex surveillance. *J Vasc Surg* 21:16-25, 1995.
5. Kraiss LW, Johansen K: Pharmacologic intervention to prevent graft failure. *Surg Clin North Am* 4:761-772, 1995.
6. Belin M, Conte MS, Donaldson MC, et al: Preferred strategies for secondary infrainguinal bypasses: Lessons learned from 300 consecutive reoperations. *J Vasc Surg* 21:282-295, 1995.
7. Donaldson MC, Whittemore AD, Mannick JA: Further experience

with an all autogenous tissue policy for infrainguinal reconstruction. *J Vasc Surg* 18:41-48, 1993.

8. Seeger JM, Pretus H, Carlton LM, et al: Predictors of outcome in patients with tissue loss undergoing infrainguinal revascularization. Presented at the 23rd annual meeting for The Southern Association of Vascular Surgery, Naples, Florida, January, 1999.

9. Shortell CK, Ouriel K, Green RM, et al: Vascular disease in the antiphospholipid syndrome: A comparison with the patient population with atherosclerosis. *J Vasc Surg* 15:158-166, 1992.

10. Clyne CA, Archer TJ, Atuhaire, et al: Random control trial of a short course of aspirin and dipyridamole for femorodistal grafts. *Br J Surg* 74:246-248, 1987.

11. Becquemin JP: Effect of ticlopidine on the long term patency of saphenous vein bypass grafts in the legs. *N Engl J Med* 337:1726-1731, 1997.

12. Rutherford RB, Jones DN, Bergentz SE, et al: The efficacy of dextran 40 in preventing early post operative graft thrombosis following difficult lower extremity bypass. *J Vasc Surg* 1:765-773, 1984.

13. Donayre CE, Ouriel K, Rhee RY, et al: Future alternatives to heparin: Low molecular weight heparin and hirudin. *J Vasc Surg* 15:675-682, 1992.

14. Sarac TP, Huber TS, Back MR, et al: Warfarin improves the outcome of infrainguinal vein bypass grafting at high risk for failure. *J Vasc Surg* 28:446-457, 1998.

15. McMillan WD, McCarthy WJ, Lin SJ, et al: Perioperative low molecular weight heparin for infrageniculate bypass. *J Vasc Surg* 25:796-802, 1997.

16. Sullivan KI, Gardner GA, Kandarpa K, et al: Efficacy of thrombolysis in infrainguinal bypass grafts. *Circulation* 83:99I-105I, 1991.

17. Antiplatelet Trialists: Collaborative overview of randomized trial of antiplatelet therapy: II. Maintenance of vascular graft or arterial patency by platelet therapy. *Br Med J* 308:159-168, 1994.

18. Leon MB, Baim DS, Popma JJ, et al: A clinical trial comparing three antithrombotic drug regimens after coronary stenting. Stent anticoagulation restenosis study investigators. *N Engl J Med* 339:1665-1671, 1998.

19. Calverley DC, Roth GJ: Antiplatelet therapy: Aspirin, ticlopidine/ clopidogrel, as anti-integrin agents. *Hematol Oncol Clin North Am* - 12:1231-1241, 1998.

20. Harward TRS, Coe D, Flynn TC, et al: The use of arm vein conduits during infrageniculate arterial vein bypass. *J Vasc Surg* 16:420-427, 1992.

21. Flinn WR, Rohrer MJ, Yao JS, et al: Improved long term patency of infragenicular polytetraethylene grafts. *J Vasc Surg* 7:685-690, 1988.

22. Kretschmer G, Herbst F, Prager M, et al: A decade of oral anticoagulant treatment to maintain autologous vein grafts for femoropopliteal atherosclerosis *Arch Surg* 127:1112-1115, 1992.

23. Arfvidsson B, Lundgren F, Drott C, et al: Influence of coumarin treatment on patency and limb salvage after peripheral arterial reconstructive surgery. *Surgery* 159:556-560, 1990.

24. Johnson WC, Blebea J, Cantelmo NL, et al: Does oral anticoagulation

improve patency of vein bypass? A prospective randomized trial. Proceedings from the 51st Annual SVS/ISCUS Meeting, Boston, 1997, (abstract p 44A).

25. Jackson MR, Claggett GP: Antithrombotic therapy in peripheral arterial occlusive disease. *Chest* 114:666S-682S, 1998.

26. Petty GW, Brown RD, Whisnant JP, et al: Frequency of major complications of aspirin, warfarin, and intravenous heparin for secondary stroke prevention. *Ann Intern Med* 130:14-22, 1999.

CHAPTER 12

Anticoagulants: Old and New

Thomas W. Wakefield, M.D.
Professor of Surgery, Section of Vascular Surgery, Department of Surgery,
University of Michigan, Ann Arbor, Michigan

This chapter will focus on anticoagulants, old and new. A discussion of the basic mechanisms of coagulation will be followed by a description of the various anticoagulants available.

BASICS OF COAGULATION

Coagulation can be described as a system with delicate balances among thrombus formation, thrombus inhibition, and physiologic fibrinolysis. An understanding of anticoagulants requires an understanding of the basic mechanism of thrombus formation. Two systems or pathways have been described: the extrinsic, or tissue factor–mediated pathway and the intrinsic pathway. It is less important today to consider two separate pathways and more important to understand that complexes of coagulation factors on activated platelet surfaces are key to thrombus formation.[1]

With injury, tissue factor binds to activated factor VII (VIIa), which activates factors IX and X to IXa and Xa. Although the enzyme responsible for the initial activation of factor VII to VIIa is unknown, factors Xa and VIIa catalyze activation of factor VII to VIIa, which amplifies the initiation of coagulation. At the same time, platelets become activated, change shape, and externalize negatively charged membranes rich in phosphatidylserine and phosphatidylinositol.[2] These membranes are key to the formation of coagulation complexes. Additionally, during platelet activation, microparticles are released that are rich in receptors for activated factors V (Va) and VIII (VIIIa). Platelets adhere to the site of injury via glycoprotein Ib (GpIb) and aggregate through fibrinogen bridging between GpIIb/IIIa receptors.

Once platelet plug formation has occurred, factors Xa, Va, ionized calcium, and factor II (prothrombin) form on the platelet surface in the prothrombinase complex, which catalyzes the conversion of prothrombin to thrombin.[1] Small amounts of formed thrombin then amplify the entire process of coagulation by (1) converting fibrinogen to fibrin, (2) activating factor XIII to XIIIa, which cross-links the fibrin clot to make it firm, (3) activating more platelets, and (4) activating factors V and VIII, two nonenzymatic cofactors, to Va and VIIIa. Additionally, small amounts of thrombin in conjunction with negatively charged surfaces[3] generate factor XIa (intrinsic pathway), which can then activate factor IX to IXa. The assembly of factors IXa, thrombin-activated VIIIa, and factor X in the presence of calcium converts factor X to Xa in the tenase complex.[1] This factor Xa can then become incorporated into more prothrombinase complexes. In this fashion, both the tissue factor–mediated pathway and the intrinsic system result in the generation of thrombin through coagulation complexes. Additionally, the

TABLE 1.
Anticoagulants and Related Compounds

Anticoagulants
    Conventional standard unfractionated heparin
    Low-molecular-weight heparin
    Danaparoid sodium
Thrombin Inhibitors
    Hirudin, Hirulog
    Argatroban
    Lepirudin
Defibrinating Agent
    Ancrod
Other Anticoagulants
    Factor X inhibitors
    Tissue factor pathway inhibitor
    Activated protein C
Antiplatelet Agents
    Aspirin, Indomethacin
    Dipyridamole
    Ticlopidine, Clopidogrel
    GpIIb/IIIa inhibitors
        -Antibodies
        -RGD mimics

Abbreviations: GpIIb/IIIa, glycoprotein IIb/IIIa; *RGD*, arginive-glycine-aspantic acid.

intrinsic system activators also can directly convert plasminogen to plasmin, thus stimulating fibrinolysis.

With the above pathophysiology of coagulation in mind, the actions of anticoagulants and related compounds can be better understood (Table 1). Heparins work through the potentiation of antithrombin III to inhibit thrombin, factor Xa, and other factors of the coagulation mechanism. As thrombin is key and central to the whole process of clot formation, direct antithrombins inhibit all the actions of thrombin, including platelet activation (accounting for their tendencies to cause bleeding). Finally, because platelet phospholipid membranes are so important for coagulation complex formation, antiplatelet agents are directed against various mechanisms of platelet activation and action.

STANDARD UNFRACTIONATED HEPARIN

Standard unfractionated heparin is a mixture of sulfated polysaccharides of varying molecular weights ranging from 2,000 to 40,000 d. Heparin is obtained from beef lung or porcine intestine. The mechanism of action of conventional unfractionated heparin includes binding to antithrombin III, which potentiates its capability to inhibit thrombin and other serine proteases of coagulation (Fig 1).[4] The half-life of unfractionated heparin is dose-dependent, that is, the greater the dose, the longer the half-life. In addition to anticoagulation, unfractionated heparin also decreases platelet aggregation in most cases. Heparin is cleared by the reticuloendothelial system, and it does not cross the placental barrier.

Clinical uses of unfractionated heparin include anticoagulation for acute arterial embolism, venous thrombosis, pulmonary embolism, and therapeutic cardiovascular procedures and prophylaxis for venous thromboembolism. The most frequent complication of heparin use is bleeding. A lower frequency of bleeding complications has been noted with continuous infusion rather than bolus infusion. The risk of bleeding is increased in the elder-

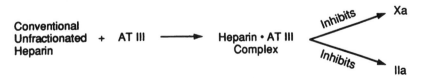

FIGURE 1.
Conventional unfractionated heparin works by augmenting the capability of antithrombin III (AT III) to inhibit factors Xa and IIa (thrombin) along with other coagulation factors. (Courtesy of Wakefield TW, Stanley JC: Interoperative heparin anticoagulation and its reversal. *Semin Vasc Surg* 9: 296-302, 1996.)

ly, in postmenopausal women, in uremic patients, and in patients with pre-existent abnormalities in platelet or coagulation function.[5] Long-term heparin usage, especially if given at a dosage of 20,000 IU/day or more for longer than 6 months, can lead to osteoporosis. Alopecia is another heparin side effect. However, the most devastating side effect is heparin-induced thrombocytopenia and the more severe heparin-induced thrombocytopenia and thrombosis syndrome (HITTS). Morbidity and mortality rates have been reported as high as approximately 60% and 20%, respectively. This syndrome is caused by a heparin-dependent IgG antibody. The antibody aggregates platelets when it is directed against the heparin-platelet factor IV (PF-4) complex. Both bovine and porcine heparin may cause this problem, and both arterial and venous thrombosis have been reported. Even the small amount of heparin present in arterial line flushes or on heparin-coated intravascular devices has been reported to cause these problems. The diagnosis is suspected when there is more than a 50% fall in platelet count during heparin therapy or a platelet count less than 100,000. Laboratory tests include the serotonin release assay—the gold standard—(sensitivity and specificity, greater than 90%), a less sensitive platelet aggregation test, and a relatively new enzyme-linked immunosorbent assay test for detection of the antibody. Because of the serious nature of this syndrome, any patient receiving heparin should have platelet counts measured beginning 3 days after heparin therapy is begun and sooner if exposed to heparin in the past.

Treatment for heparin-induced thrombocytopenia consists of stopping heparin and using another anticoagulant. Although plasmapheresis, platelet apheresis, and IV immunoglobulin were suggested in the past, pharmacologic approaches are recommended today. As patients with this syndrome demonstrate circulating platelet microparticles, they have a heightened thrombotic risk, and warfarin administration initially can potentiate this risk. Thus, warfarin must be begun under the protection of another anticoagulant. Available alternative anticoagulants include low-molecular weight heparins (LMWHs), although cross-reactivity in our laboratory is more than 90%, and unless a LMWH tests negative in vitro, it should not be substituted. Danaparoid sodium (Orgaran), a heparinoid, has approximately a 20% to 25% risk of cross-reactivity and is a better choice. Antiplatelet agents such as aspirin and glycoprotein IIb/IIIa receptor antagonists have been suggested, as has ancrod (Arvin), a defibrinating agent that requires 12 hours to achieve acceptable levels for anticoagulation. The best choices today are direct thrombin inhibitors, such as argatroban (Novastan) and lepirudin (Refludan), which has recently been approved for this use by the Food and Drug Administration. Lepirudin, a recombinant derivative of hirudin, is excreted in the urine and has a half-life of 1.3 hours. It is given intravenously and is followed using activated partial thromboplastin times (aPTTs).[6] With early diagnosis and aggressive appropriate treatment, morbidity and mortality rates as low as 7.4% and 1.1%, respectively, have been achieved.[7]

LOW-MOLECULAR WEIGHT HEPARIN

LMWH preparations were developed to decrease the risk of bleeding from standard unfractionated heparin. LMWHs are composed of the lower molecular weight range of standard heparin preparations, and, as such, the anticoagulant mechanisms are different. Standard unfractionated heparin is capable of inhibiting thrombin because it is large enough to make a three-way complex between itself, thrombin, and antithrombin III. LMWH preparations are mostly not large enough to make this complex and thus have less antithrombin activity. A minimum chain length of 18 saccharide units is necessary for formation of this ternary complex. However, to inhibit factor Xa, such a ternary complex is not necessary; thus, LMWHs are capable of inhibiting factor Xa (Fig 2). In fact, each LMWH has its own ratio of antifactor Xa to antifactor IIa (thrombin) activity, depending on its size and molecular weight. Most commercially available LMWHs have ratios between 4:1 and 2:1, whereas standard unfractionated heparin has a 1:1 ratio.[8] Because the bleeding potential of heparin is believed to be related, in large part, to its antithrombin activity, LMWHs should have a lower bleeding potential. Additionally, LMWHs are believed to have less antiplatelet activity and a lower risk for HIT and HITTS.

LMWHs have other advantages over standard unfractionated heparin, including an improved pharmacokinetic profile due to reduced nonspecific binding to plasma proteins, less lipolysis, a non–dose-dependent half-life, more constant antifactor Xa inhibition, less interference with protein C activation, a decrease in com-

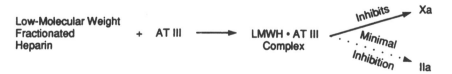

FIGURE 2.
Low-molecular weight heparin (LMWH) potentiates the capability of antithrombin III (AT III) to inhibit more factor Xa than IIa (thrombin) because of the small size of LMWH. (Courtesy of Wakefield TW, Stanley JC: Interoperative heparin anticoagulation and its reversal. *Semin Vasc Surg* 9: 296-302, 1996.)

plement activation, less interference with appropriate platelet aggregation, less risk for osteoporosis, and a lower level of fibrin monomer production.[8] High and sustained plasma antifactor Xa levels exist for greater than 16 hours after administration of LMWH in therapeutic doses, and excretion is primarily renal. However, there is no agent available today effective for LMWH reversal as measured by antifactor Xa levels.

LMWHs were first used in deep venous thrombosis (DVT) prophylaxis, and they have become the prophylactic agent of choice in orthopedic hip and knee surgery and in high-risk patients undergoing general surgery.[9] More recently, these agents have been used in the full treatment of DVT and pulmonary embolism. A number of studies and two meta-analyses have compared LMWH with standard unfractionated heparin in the treatment of DVT.[10,11] In aggregate, these studies suggest a lower risk of major bleeding, a lower risk of recurrent thromboembolic disease, and a lower risk of death than standard unfractionated heparin. Even for pulmonary embolism, LMWH appears at least equivalent to standard unfractionated heparin but much more convenient.[12] It is not necessary to monitor LMWH with coagulation testing except in specific situations such as renal failure, and most regimens use either fixed-dose or weight-adjusted dosing given subcutaneously. Because of the lack of need for frequent coagulation testing, outpatient treatment has been demonstrated in several trials. However, a number of different services need to be coordinated for such outpatient treatment to be successful, including home nursing, pharmacy, coagulation (for warfarin monitoring), and physician services.

The economic impact of the use of LMWH rather than standard unfractionated heparin for the treatment of venous thromboembolism has been investigated. Cost savings have ranged from greater than $300,000 for 125 patients (or approximately $2,400 per case) in the United States[13] to approximately $4,000 U.S. dollars per case in Canada[14] and to a more than 60% reduction in costs in a study involving centers in Europe, Australia, and New Zealand.[15] Additionally, once-per-day treatment with LMWH (dalteparin) resulted in large cost reductions in a large multicenter Swedish study.[16] Expanded indications for treatment—withholding LMWH treatment only from those with massive pulmonary embolism, a high risk for major or active bleeding, or phlegmasia and from patients already hospitalized for other diseases—have resulted in greater than 80% of patients becoming eligible for outpatient treatment.[17] Furthermore, some 90% of these patients report high satisfaction with home outpatient treatment.[18]

LMWH has also been studied in unstable angina.[8] LMWH has been found to be superior to a placebo and equivalent or superior to standard unfractionated heparin in terms of the end points of death or myocardial infarction, without any increase in major bleeding. The question remains whether one preparation of LMWH will be found superior to another or whether all preparations will share the same advantages for the treatment of DVT, pulmonary embolism, and unstable angina.

OTHER ANTICOAGULANTS
HIRUDIN
Hirudin, which is obtained from the saliva of leeches, is a single-chain polypeptide. It is composed of 65 amino acids, has a molecular weight of 8,000 to 9,000 d, and has three disulfide bonds. Hirudin has a short half-life of 15 to 30 minutes and is excreted in the urine. It is a direct inhibitor of thrombin and opposes all of thrombin's actions, including conversion of fibrinogen to fibrin, activation of factors V, VIII, and XIII to Va, VIIIa, and XIIIa, respectively, and thrombin-induced platelet aggregation.[19] Hirudin is more potent than heparin in reducing platelet deposition and mural thrombosis at similar aPTT levels. Hirudin also prevents the growth of thrombi at high and low shear rates of blood flow and can stop the growth of thrombi, even in severe stenoses. Unlike heparin, which can inhibit only free, circulating unbound thrombin, hirudin and other direct thrombin inhibitors act against both circulating thrombin and clot-bound thrombin. The high incidence of bleeding from hirudin, however, limits its usefulness clinically.[20] The gene for hirudin was cloned in 1986, which led the way to the recombinant production of analogues such as Hirulog and lepirudin. Hirulog is much less potent than hirudin and reveals an apparent lack of toxicity and immunogencity.[20] Argatroban (a synthetic organic antithrombin) has been found useful for the treatment of patients with HIT and HITTS. In addition, lepirudin has now been FDA approved for use in HIT and HITTS and has an acceptable bleeding profile.

ANCROD
Ancrod is another alternative anticoagulant, and its use during infrainguinal bypass surgery has been reported.[21] This is a thrombin-like enzyme derived from the Malayan pit viper. Ancrod produces a controlled decrease in fibrinogen levels by depleting fibrinopeptide A, but not fibrinopeptide B, from fibrinogen. The fibrin monomers that result stimulate the local production of tissue plasminogen activator. Both of these actions lead to a state of anticoagulation. However, the level of fibrinogen must be closely monitored to prevent bleeding. Other agents that are being developed against various aspects of the coagulation system include factor X

inhibitors, tissue factor pathway inhibitor, and activated protein C.[2] Platelet aggregation is another target for inhibition.

ANTIPLATELET AGENTS

Platelet aggregation can be inhibited by (1) blocking cyclooxygenase, the first step in the conversion of arachidonic acid to thromboxane A_2, (2) blocking thromboxane synthase, the enzyme leading to the production of thromboxane A_2, (3) blocking the thromboxane A_2 receptor, (4) increasing the intraplatelet levels of cyclic adenosine monophosphate (cAMP) or cyclic guanosine monophosphate, which inhibit the exposure of the platelet GpIIb/IIIa receptor, or (5) directly blocking the GpIIb/IIIa receptor. Aspirin and indomethacin inhibit cyclooxygenase, thus inhibiting both prostacyclin and thromboxane, whereas methylxanthines such as dipyridamole (Persantine) inhibit phosphodiesterase, which leads to higher levels of cAMP. Ticlopidine interferes with platelet aggregation, mediated by adenosine diphosphate. Because of ticlopidine-associated neutropenia, a ticlopidine analogue, clopidogrel, was developed. This thienopyridine compound is not associated with the same degree of neutropenia and has been shown to reduce the composite end points of a stroke, myocardial infarction, and death in patients with vascular disease.[2]

Direct inhibitors of GpIIb/IIIa were first developed as murine-derived monoclonal antibodies. The compound abciximab (C7E3Fab; ReoPro) is a chimeric antibody form of the monoclonal antibody directed at the GpIIb/IIIa receptor and is the first agent of this class to be clinically available.[2] Its receptor binding is non-specific, and it binds to other cell-surface integrins. Agents in development include anginine-glycine-aspantic acid mimics that act as competitive antagonists to the GpIIb/IIIa receptor, including the cyclic peptide eptifibatide (Integrilin), the parenteral nonpeptide mimetics lamifiban and tirofiban (Aggrastat), the oral nonpeptide mimetics xemilofiban, orbofiban, roxifiban, sibrafiban, lefradafiban, and SB 214857, and the parenteral and oral nonpeptide mimetic RPR-109891 (Klerval).[22] Most studies with these agents have involved coronary interventions, unstable angina, or myocardial infarction, in which these agents have shown an advantage.[2] The use of these agents in peripheral vascular interventions will require rigorous future study.

REFERENCES

1. Hassouna HI: Laboratory evaluation of hemostatic disorders, in Penner JA, Hassouna HI (eds): *Coagulation Disorders II. Hematology/Oncology Clinics of North America.* Philadelphia, W.B. Saunders Company, 1993, pp 1161-1249.

2. Ferguson JJ, Waly HM, Wilson JM: Fundamentals of coagulation and glycoprotein IIb/IIIa receptor inhibition. *Eur Heart J* 19:D3S-D9S, 1998.
3. Naito K, Fujikawa K: Activation of human blood coagulation factor XI independent of factor XII. Factor XI is activated by thrombin and factor XIa in the presence of negatively charged surfaces. *J Biol Chem* 266:7353-7358, 1991.
4. Hirsh J: Heparin. *N Engl J Med* 324:1565-1574, 1991.
5. Wakefield TW, Stanley JC: Intraoperative heparin anticoagulation and its reversal. *Semin Vasc Surg* 9:296-302, 1996.
6. Lepirudin for heparin-induced thrombocytopenia. *Med Lett* 40:94-95, 1998.
7. Almeida JI, Coats R, Liem TK, et al: Reduced morbidity and mortality rates of the heparin-induced thrombocytopenia syndrome. *J Vasc Surg* 27:309-316, 1998.
8. Hirsh J: Low-molecular-weight heparin: A review of the results of recent studies of the treatment of venous thromboembolism and unstable angina. *Circulation* 98:1575-1582, 1998.
9. Clagett GP, Anderson FA Jr, Heit J, et al: Prevention of venous thromboembolism. *Chest* 108:312S-334S, 1995.
10. Leizorovicz A: Comparison of the efficacy and safety of low molecular weight heparins and unfractionated heparin in the initial treatment of deep venous thrombosis: An updated meta-analysis. *Drugs* 52(Suppl 7):30S-37S, 1996.
11. Siragusa S, Cosmi B, Piovella F, et al: Low-molecular-weight heparins and unfractionated heparin in the treatment of patients with acute venous thromboembolism: Results of a meta-analysis. *Am J Med* 100:269-277, 1996.
12. Simonneau G, Sors H, Charbonnier B, et al: A comparison of low-molecular-weight heparin with unfractionated heparin for acute pulmonary embolism. The THESEE study group. *N Engl J Med* 337:663-669, 1997.
13. Groce JB III: Patient outcomes and cost analysis associated with an outpatient deep venous thrombosis treatment program. *Pharmacotherapy* 18:175S-180S, 1998.
14. Hull RD, Raskob GE, Rosenbloom D, et al: Treatment of proximal vein thrombosis with subcutaneous low-molecular-weight heparin vs intravenous heparin: An economic perspective. *Arch Intern Med* 157:289-294, 1997.
15. van den Belt AG, Bossuyt PM, Prins MH, et al: Replacing inpatient care by outpatient care in the treatment of deep venous thrombosis—An economic evaluation. Tasman Study Group *Thromb Haemost* 79:259-263, 1998.
16. Lindmarker P, Holmstrom M: Use of low-molecular-weight heparin (dalteparin), once daily, for the treatment of deep vein thrombosis: A feasibility and health economic study in an outpatient setting. Swedish Venous Thrombosis Doltepanin Trial Group *J Intern Med* 240:395-401, 1996.
17. Wells PS, Kovacs MJ, Bormanis J, et al: Expanding eligibility for out-

patient treatment of deep venous thrombosis and pulmonary embolism with low-molecular-weight heparin: A comparison of patient self-injection with homecare injection. *Arch Intern Med* 158:1809-1812, 1998.

18. Harrison L, McGinnis J, Crowther M, et al: Assessment of outpatient treatment of deep-vein thrombosis with low-molecular-weight heparin. *Arch Intern Med* 158:2001-2003, 1998.

19. Hull RD, Pineo GF, Raskob GE: Hirudin versus heparin and low-molecular-weight heparin: And the winner is.... *J Lab Clin Med* 132:171-174, 1998.

20. Fenton JW III, Ofosu FA, Brezniak DV, et al: Thrombin and antithrombotics. *Semin Thromb Hemost* 24:87-91, 1998.

21. Cole CW, Bormanis J, Luna GK, et al: Ancrod versus heparin for anticoagulation during surgical procedures. *J Vasc Surg* 17:288-293, 1993.

22. Madan M, Berkowitz SD, Tcheng JE: Glycoprotein IIb/IIIa integrin blockade. *Circulation* 98:2629-2635, 1998.

PART V
Imaging Techniques

CHAPTER 13

Duplex Three-Dimensional Ultrasound: Potential Benefits

E. John Harris, Jr., M.D.
Assistant Professor of Surgery, Division of Vascular Surgery, Stanford University School of Medicine, Stanford, California; Medical Director, Stanford Vascular Laboratory

The ultimate goal of noninvasive vascular imaging is to provide an accurate yet easily visualized image of the vascular structure interrogated. Because of its low cost and high utility, US has become the predominant tool for noninvasive vascular imaging. Transmitting an acoustic wave into the body using an ultrasonic transducer and interpreting the waves that are reflected back to the transducer creates US images. The character of the returning waves is dependent on the interaction of the transmitted wave with the tissue it enters. Physical parameters influencing this interaction include the speed of sound in tissue, the attenuation coefficient of the US wave, and the acoustic impedance of the tissue being imaged. Attenuation refers to loss of energy of the wave in traveling through the tissue and is related to absorption and scattering of the US energy. Acoustic impedance represents the different reflections of US waves at different tissue interfaces, which influences the image quality of US.

Early use of US in noninvasive vascular imaging involved the carotid artery. When satisfactory images were obtained, estimates of plaque morphological features were accurate, but estimates of percent stenosis were not accurate for more than mild stenoses. It is often difficult to estimate the size of the arterial lumen from a B-mode image alone because the interface between the arterial wall and flowing blood is not clearly seen.

Conventional US is two-dimensional (2-D) as currently used, requiring the investigator to view multiple tomographic images and then collate these images into a mental picture of a true three-dimensional (3-D) structure. Currently, 2-D real-time US imaging is a safe and relatively cheap method of vascular imaging. There are, however, several drawbacks of 2-D US imaging compared with other imaging methods such as CT and MRI. These limitations include the low signal-to-noise ratio of US images, the inability of US to pass through air or bone, nonuniform spatial resolutions of US images, and the lack of 3-D US images.

DEVELOPMENT OF DUPLEX US

Pulsed Doppler signals were added to B-mode imaging to create the "duplex," a technique developed in the 1970s, in an effort to improve the US detection of arterial stenoses. The severity of the stenosis was graded on the basis of information obtained from the spectral waveform analysis of the Doppler signal. The spectral waveform criteria for classifying the severity of carotid arterial stenoses have been validated in several centers of excellence by comparison against independently interpreted arteriograms, with specificities greater than 85% and sensitivities of 99%. The accuracy for detecting 50% to 99% stenosis or occlusion with these validated criteria approaches 95%.

A problem experienced with duplex scanning has been operator variability; skilled technicians could duplicate these results, whereas novice technicians could not. Placing the pulsed Doppler sample volume in the area of most disturbed flow was critical to the accuracy of the test and required skill not only in imaging the target vessel but also in interpreting the audio signal for acquisition of the optimal sample site (volume). This weakness was significantly improved by the addition of color flow imaging techniques developed in the 1980s.

In contrast to spectral analysis, which evaluates the entire frequency and amplitude content of the signal at a single sample site, color flow imaging provides a simultaneous estimate of the Doppler-shifted frequencies or flow velocities within the entire B-mode image. Spectral waveforms contain a range of frequencies and amplitudes, allowing determination of flow direction and spectral parameters such as mean, mode, peak, and bandwidth. The color assignments in color flow imaging are based on flow and a single mean frequency estimate for each site in the B-mode image plane. Therefore, a visual real-time clue to the area of highest flow velocity is possible with less operator variability, and this site of maximal velocity can then be sampled for spectral analysis for determination of the degree of stenosis. Variations in Doppler-shifted frequency or flow velocities are then indicated by changes in color, and lighter colors typically represent higher flow velocities.

Color flow imaging has its own limitations. Random noise in color flow imaging obscures low-level Doppler signals, which makes detection of slow flow a problem. As with duplex Doppler, color flow imaging signals are dependent on the angle at which the US beam intersects the direction of blood flow. The most accuracy comes with an angle of insonation approaching 0 degrees. As the angle of insonation approaches 90 degrees, the Doppler-shifted frequencies drop to zero, thus giving the appearance of no flow. In practice, because of the anatomy of the neck, the angle of insonation is usually close to 60 degrees.

Color Doppler energy (CDE) imaging has recently been developed to address some of these problems. In CDE imaging, the US system calculates the energy of the returning Doppler signal rather than its mean frequency or velocity. CDE imaging is angle independent; as the angle of insonation changes, there is little change in the total energy of the Doppler signal. Therefore, CDE imaging can detect flow in vessels at a right angle to the US beam. In CDE imaging, low-flow signals are less likely to be obscured by noise than in color flow imaging. Because the energy of the background noise is significantly lower than the energy of the blood flow signal, the background noise is represented as a homogeneous background against which the blood vessel is sharply contrasted. However, CDE imaging does not provide information on the speed or direction of blood flow: flow is either present or not. Subtle soft-tissue motion can also create a flash artifact in CDE imaging. Currently, carotid artery noninvasive evaluation relies on color flow duplex imaging with occasional use of the CDE component.

B-mode US imaging has improved considerably during its 40-year lifetime. Most of the recent improvements in image quality are not due to any new physical properties but rather to the rapid improvements in electronic and computing technologies. High-speed digital processing is spearheading the current improvements, allowing beam formation and signal processing to occur with ever-increasing precision and flexibility. Digital processing also significantly decreases scanning times, which is critical to real-time US. In spite of these advances, the transducer sets the fundamental performance limits of any US scanner, and exciting innovations in transducer technology are just now being realized. New innovations using variable or larger transducer bandwidths, parallel US beam forming, dynamic and spatial filtering, and improved phase array technologies have and will continue to improve image quality. Although current high-quality B-mode images, augmented with color Doppler data, are capable of providing useful information about plaque location and morphological features, the individual image viewing area is currently limited.

Without an objective 3-D image, key anatomical or pathologic features of vascular structures may be missed with this 2-D US image. Conventional 2-D US images represent only a thin slice of the particular structure at a single location and orientation, which may be difficult to reproduce at a later time. The development of an objective 3-D image of vascular structures and their lesion distributions with US images will represent an important step forward in the evolution of duplex US and noninvasive vascular imaging. A 3-D US imaging process will involve the acquisition of a set of serial or nonserial 2-D US images and subsequent reconstruction, rendering, and volumetric analysis of the entire data set. This chapter will briefly outline the progress in the development of a 3-D US process, acknowledge the main limitations of current methods, and suggest several areas for further investigation and refinement.

DEVELOPMENT OF A SYSTEM

The optimal 3-D US system will have several requirements: (1) The system should have real-time capability, (2) 2-D US scanning equipment should be used without irretrievable modifications, and (3) the freehand interactive technique should be maintained. Ideally, the image quality of 3-D images should surpass those of 2-D source images, and a 3-D US data set should be compatible with other 3-D image data sets to allow direct comparison and contrast with available 3-D image analysis software. The technician should maintain control of the location and orientation of the transducer probe and control of both the scanning and echo signal processing parameters. Color flow Doppler and CDE data displayed on top of a B-mode image may provide useful contrast.

3-D imaging of the vasculature with US is currently in its early phase of development, and several different strategies are utilized. Systems have been described for echocardiography, intravascular US, and peripheral vascular US. All systems developed for these different applications are similar in that they share the tomographic nature of US imaging. These systems vary in the manner in which these serial 2-D ultrasonic tomograms are captured and spatially oriented into a 3-D image. Video data from the US system display are converted into a 2-D image intensity array by a frame grabber. Image intensity is measured in pixels (picture elements). Because a pixel (picture element) defines a point in 2-D space with its x and y coordinates, a third z coordinate is needed.

Each 2-D image plane of a structure obtained by the US transducer can be placed into a 3-D volume. The 3-D volume is represented by x-, y-, and z-axes. There can be rotation and translation along each axis. A voxel (volume element) is a unit of graphic information that defines a point in 3-D space.

An unrestricted US probe has six degrees of freedom of movement: three rotational and three translational. The most common approach to scanning a 3-D volume with 2-D image slices is to constrain the movement of the probe to one degree of freedom. This can be produced by internal motors rotating the transducer within a mechanically fixed probe or by mechanical arms translating the probe along a fixed axis. As the probe is moved with one degree of freedom, the image plane sweeps through the volume. The area of the 2-D image and the range of movement along the one degree of freedom determine the size of the swept volume. Scanning in this manner can produce three different shapes of swept volumes, using a sector-shaped 2-D image (Fig 1).

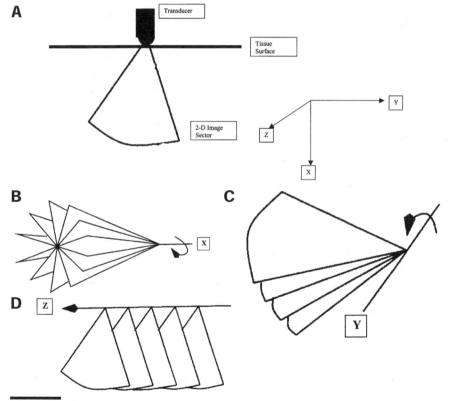

FIGURE 1.
A, a typical image plane generated by a two-dimensional (2-D) duplex US transducer. **B**, rotation of the transducer about the x-axis will generate a cone-shaped swept volume. **C**, rotation of the probe about the y-axis will generate a fan-shaped swept volume. **D**, translation of the transducer along the z-axis will generate a prism-shaped swept volume.

A cone-shaped swept volume is obtained by rotating the probe about the x-axis. A fan shaped swept volume will be produced with rotation about the y-axis. If the probe is translated along the z-axis, a prismatic swept volume is generated. The main advantage of the cone-shaped and fan-shaped data sets is the use of a small acoustic window for the entire volume sweep. Acoustic windows on the human body are often small and difficult to obtain. This method is useful for applications such as echocardiography. In practice, fixed translation of a transducer along one axis is difficult because of the curvatures experienced in human surface anatomy. Prismatic sampling has been used successfully with intravascular US because fixed translation of the probe along the axis of the blood vessel is easily accomplished. Cross-sectional images in the x and y planes are obtained and then serially stacked as the catheter is withdrawn along the z plane. Limitations common to all three of these methods are a relatively slow acquisition rate, the need for modified US transducers, and insonation from one direction only for the structure interrogated.

The simplest approach to 3-D US reconstruction from multiple 2-D image slices is to allow free motion of the US transducer. With this freehand approach, the skill of the technician is maximized. The technician is allowed to image the 3-D structure in the planes available for interrogation, which maximizes data acquisition. When a freehand approach is used, the scan planes through a region of interest are chosen by the technician to avoid areas of acoustic shadowing. Sampling a region of interest from multiple views can thus fill in a region obscured by acoustic shadowing in one isolated view. Unlike prism, fan, and cone volume scanning, which can acquire images at high speed because of high-speed motors moving the probe, freehand volume scanning is slow and decreases the possibility for real-time 3-D reconstructions. Because of motion artifacts from breathing and cardiac motion, these images are frequently gated to the cardiac cycle via a continuous ECG monitor. This cardiac gating synchronizes data acquisition to the same phase of the cardiac cycle.

SPATIAL ORIENTATION

Spatial orientation of the multiple 2-D image slices is critical to accurate 3-D reconstruction. Methods used for transducer localization and orientation have included mechanical arms, multiposition tripods, acoustic triangulation systems, laser optic triangulation systems, and magnetic field pulse-flux monitors. Calibration is required to determine the offset of the position sensor to the scan plane of the transducer. The 2-D intensity array generated by the transducer for each image plane must then be stored in a computer with the associated position data generated from the position sensor.

The same region in a 3-D structure may be sampled with 2-D images from more than one view, yet it is also possible that some areas of the structure will not be sampled. Multiple images of the same region can be compounded to decrease artifacts. Compounding occurs when pixels from multiple planes are reprojected through the same voxel; thus, compounding requires precise image registration. The entire volume cross-section does not need to appear in every image. This allows the technician imaging the structure to focus on specific regions of interest. Unlike the artifacts produced by other tomographic imaging methods, the areas of acoustic shadowing observed with US do not compromise the adjacent well-visualized areas of the volume. Compounding images from different perspectives can reduce noise artifacts but may also blur the object of interest.

THREE-DIMENSIONAL VOLUME VISUALIZATION

Volume data are represented in 3-D format through the use of visualization algorithms, which convert the stacked 2-D images into a 3-D structure. The two most common techniques for visualizing volume data are surface rendering and volume rendering. Surface rendering uses original data such as the voxel and places them within a segmentation algorithm. Surface normals are usually calculated from geometric primitives such as polygons or cubes, and voxel data are categorized into thresholds based on intensity. Then geometric primitives are automatically fit to the high-contrast contours in the volume that match the threshold. Changing the surface fit threshold value is time-consuming because each cell must be revisited to extract a new set of surface primitives for the new threshold. The segmentation process to decide whether each voxel in the data set belongs to the object is complex, and often, small details are lost or artifacts are introduced into the object.

With US data, the intensities of different tissues are similarly represented in the image, and only the interface between different tissues is visible. When an US beam passes through an object of interest, it is the interface between tissues that causes the US to be reflected. Bone and air interfaces reflect 99% of the US beam, which creates clearly visible interfaces. Within the object of interest, different tissue interfaces based on variable US wave reflections are chosen as the edge to generate surface contours; however, these differences are minimal—in most settings, they create noise within the data. The presence of noise in the data severely affects the quality of the segmentation process in the surface rendering algorithms.

Volume rendering methods involve mapping voxels directly into screen space without using geometric primitives as intermediate representation. Each element in the volume contributes color or brightness to the final 3-D image. The entire data set must be sampled each time a new 3-D image is rendered. Comparison of the color or contrast of all voxels between the current voxel and the image plane determines the amount of color or contrast contributed by a voxel. Each voxel's contribution to the image can then be calculated and composited using a series of lookup tables. The 3-D image is extracted from the data set for display using different thresholds of intensity or color. Different visualization methods of sampling the voxels in volume rendering techniques include ray-casting, volume ray-tracing, any-plane slicing, and splattering.

PRELIMINARY DEVELOPMENT AT STANFORD

The intent of our 3-D US project was to design a freehand 3-D US system based on a high spatial and contrast resolution low-noise color duplex US machine. The transducer was chosen to provide the highest frequency probe that could image to the typical depth of the carotid artery. An accurate position sensor with a high acquisition rate was necessary, and it had to be attached as close as possible to the scanning surface of the transducer. The 2-D images were acquired at close intervals to reduce gaps and aliasing. Multiple views of the same region were obtained to test compounding.

Our freehand 3-D duplex US system is based on the Hewlett-Packard HP 8500 GP US system. A 7.5-MHz linear array probe has been fitted with a pulse-flux magnetometer position locating system. The position locating system consists of a receiver mounted on the transducer head, a transmitter mounted remotely on the examining table, and a system control unit. The transmitter emits three orthogonal magnetic fields corresponding to the x, y, and z planes. The system control unit transforms position and orientation data from the receiver on the transducer into matrix form.

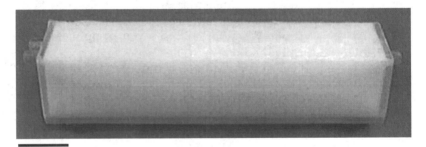

FIGURE 2.
The flow phantom has a bifurcated vessel within a tissue-mimic agar. The tissue mimic was chosen to allow US and MRI.

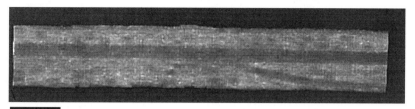

FIGURE 3.
Coronal view of three-dimensional US reconstruction of flow phantom.

These matrix data are synchronized with the 2-D duplex US image at each position. These oriented duplex data sets are transferred to a Hewlett-Packard personal computer where a proprietary visualizer (Spectrum Visualizer, Centric Engineering Systems, Inc., Santa Clara, Calif) is used to perform volume rendering of the data and a 3-D image is created. Calibration of this system against MRI data has been performed with a carotid artery flow phantom that is compatible with both US and MRI (Fig 2). A typical 3-D image from this phantom in the coronal plane is illustrated in Figure 3. The flow phantom has been used to calibrate the 3-D reconstruction process against the known dimensions of the phantom and against the data generated by 3-D reconstructions of the MRI data sets. This work and further in vivo imaging with the system is ongoing.

POTENTIAL APPLICATIONS FOR THREE-DIMENSIONAL US

Imaging of calcified plaques may be improved by allowing multiple views around the calcific shadowing. Current duplex US often cannot accurately interrogate regions of arterial wall that are heavily calcified, even though the entire circumference of the wall is not always calcified. A 3-D US system could use multiple looks to generate a view of the area obscured by calcium in one plane from the compounded images obtained in alternative planes.

Early vascular luminal lesions could potentially be detected by 3-D US volume measurements. Currently, duplex US can identify plaque within the vessel before there is hemodynamic significance to the plaque. Unfortunately, the same 2-D image plane is hard to reproduce with 2-D imaging on multiple evaluations. 3-D US would not depend on obtaining the exact same 2-D view for follow-up, and calculation of luminal volumes of a vessel from the 3-D US could be followed for disease progression with little variability. Such volume measurements could prove useful in following angioplasty restenosis rates, vein graft intimal hyperplasia progression, and intravascular stent intimal hyperplasia progression. If real-time 3-D reconstructions are realized, 3-D US may also decrease scanning times for time-consuming examinations such as carotid duplex imaging, vein graft flow velocity studies, and venous insufficiency examinations.

Perforator localization could be greatly enhanced by a 3-D US examination. A 3-D rendering of perforator locations and incompetent superficial valve sites would be invaluable for surgical approaches to venous insufficiency. It is possible that a duplex transducer coupled to a 3-D US system could be used in real time to localize incompetent perforators for the subfascial endoscopic perforator surgery-type procedures now requiring extensive preoperative mapping.

A 3-D US system would also be useful in following endovascular stent grafts used for treatment of abdominal aortic aneurysms. The volume of the aneurysmal sac could be followed to monitor exclusion of the aneurysm, and any endoleaks that developed could be localized, all at a significantly decreased risk and cost compared with CT scans, which are currently used.

SUGGESTED READING

Zierler RE: Carotid artery evaluation by duplex scanning. *Semin Vasc Surg* 1:9-16, 1988.

Zierler RE, Phillips DJ, Beach KW, et al: Noninvasive assessment of normal carotid bifurcation hemodynamics with color-flow US imaging. *US Med Biol* 13:471-476, 1987.

Fenster A, Lee D, Sherebin S, et al: Three-dimensional US imaging of the vasculature. *Ultrasonics* 36:629-633, 1998.

Hodges TC, Detmer PR, Burns DH, et al: Ultrasonic three-dimensional reconstruction: In vitro and in vivo volume and area measurement. *US Med Biol* 20:719-729, 1994.

Pretorius DH, Nelson TR, Jaffe JS: 3-Dimensional sonographic analysis based on color flow Doppler and gray scale image data: A preliminary report. *J US Med* 11:225-232, 1992.

Rankin RN, Fenster A, Downey DB, et al: Three-dimensional sonographic reconstruction: Techniques and diagnostic applications. *AJR Am J Roentgenol* 161:695-702, 1993.

Barry CD, Allott CP, John NW, et al: Three-dimensional freehand US: Image reconstruction and volume analysis. *US Med Biol* 23:1209-1224, 1997.

Nelson TR, Elvins TT: Visualization of 3D US data. *IEEE Comput Graph Appl* 13:50-57, 1993.

Whittingham TA: New and future developments in US imaging. *Br J Radiol* 70:119S-132S, 1997.

Prager RW, Rohling RN, Gee AH, et al: Rapid calibration for 3-D freehand US. *US Med Biol* 24:855-869, 1998.

Rohling RN, Gee AH, Berman L: Automatic registration of 3-D US images. *US Med Biol* 24:841-854, 1998.

PART VI
Portal Hypertension

C HAPTER 14

Transjugular Intrahepatic Portosystemic Shunts

David P. Brophy, M.D.
Assistant Professor of Radiology, Harvard Medical School, Boston,
Massachusetts; Cardiovascular and Interventional Radiologist,
Department of Radiology, Beth Israel Deaconess Medical Center, Boston,
Massachusetts

Laura J. Perry, M.D.
Instructor of Radiology, Harvard Medical School, Boston, Massachusetts;
Angiographer and Interventional Radiologist, Department of Radiology,
Beth Israel Deaconess Medical Center, Boston, Massachusetts

L ife-threatening recurrent variceal hemorrhaging and intractable
ascites are known consequences of portal venous hypertension
and cirrhosis. First-line medical management has consisted of
drug therapy to lower portal pressure (e.g., octreotide acetate, anti-
hypertensives, and IV vasopressin), sodium restriction and repeated paracentesis to control ascites, and endoscopic sclerosis and
banding of bleeding varices. Traditionally, patients in whom the
aforementioned measures failed were offered definitive treatment
with an open surgical portosystemic shunt. Although surgically
created portosystemic bypasses have a very high technical and
clinical success rate and are lasting, the frequent urgent nature of
the procedure and concurrent mesenteric and other abdominal
varices can make the operation difficult and potentially complicated. An emergent surgical shunt can have a mortality rate of
more than 50%, usually because of bleeding complications.[1] Liver
transplantation might be considered the ultimate "cure" for these
patients, but this alternative is limited by donor availability.

First described in 1982 by Colapinto et al.,[2] transjugular intrahepatic portosystemic shunting (TIPS) is a minimally invasive
interventional radiologic procedure. The tract (shunt) through the
liver parenchyma (intrahepatic) between a portal vein (porto-) and

a hepatic vein (systemic) is created percutaneously through the transjugular route and is reinforced with a metal mesh stent. In 1969, when Rosch et al.[3] originally performed this procedure in dogs, the tracts were created with an angioplasty balloon alone, without leaving in any permanent scaffold across the vascular connection. Therefore, although portal decompression was realized in the short term, the parenchymal shunts occluded fairly rapidly. Advances in equipment technology allowed percutaneous placement of balloon-expandable and self-expanding metal stents, greatly improving shunt patency. Animal laboratory trials of TIPS with metal stents were reported by Palmaz et al.[4] (1985) and Rosch et al.[5] (1987), confirming feasibility, safety, and efficacy. In 1989, the first case of TIPS use in a human was described in the English literature by Richter et al.,[6] followed by a series of nine patients reported by the same authors in 1990.[7] Since that time, more than 30,000 TIPS procedures have been performed internationally, and some centers have completed more than 70 procedures annually.

TIPS is now accepted as an established treatment in the control of acute variceal bleeding resistant to sclerotherapy and/or banding. In addition, TIPS has been shown to be effective in alleviating intractable ascites and/or hepatic hydrothorax in patients with cirrhosis and has been applied as a bridge to planned orthotopic liver transplantation.[8,9]

INDICATIONS AND CONTRAINDICATIONS

The most well-established and frequent indication for TIPS is in the management of gastroesophageal variceal bleeding, uncontrolled by repeated sclerotherapy or inaccessible endoscopically. In this setting, TIPS may be needed urgently or emergently. Patients with cirrhosis and ileostomies or colostomies who have recurrent peristomal variceal bleeding can also be successfully treated with TIPS. Similarly, bleeding anorectal varices respond to TIPS decompression. Hemorrhaging from portal hypertensive gastropathy has been controlled with TIPS when less invasive management fails.

TIPS is also now accepted as effective in treating patients with massive intractable ascites or disabling recurrent hydrothorax ("hepatic hydrothorax"), which occurs in approximately 10% of patients with cirrhosis. The decision to create a percutaneous shunt in a patient after failed maximized conservative therapy is based on patient discomfort, respiratory compromise, lifestyle limitations, and if there has been an unacceptably short interval between taps.

Other factors to be considered when contemplating assignment of a given patient to TIPS vs. other treatment include patient compliance, geographic proximity to medical care, and insight on the part of the patient and family. Can the patient tolerate the risk of recurrent bleeding for the weeks required to complete sclerotherapy and is the patient expected to cooperate with return visits? Is the patient compliant with medications, dietary restrictions, and alcohol avoidance? Is the patient expected to return for mandatory shunt surveillance? Does the patient live in an area remote from adequate medical care or have problems with transportation? Is liver transplantation ultimately an option?

Contraindications to TIPS include severe liver failure and poorly controlled encephalopathy, as the shunt will further divert portal flow away from the liver. Hepatic blood flow decreases an estimated 20% to 30% with a successful shunt[10,11] and progressive liver failure is a rare but understandable possible outcome after TIPS. Moderate-to-severe encephalopathy can worsen after TIPS for the same reason.

Because performance of TIPS results in a rather abrupt and significant increase in already hyperdynamic circulation, the procedure is contraindicated in those with right-sided heart compromise or pulmonary hypertension. Patients with constrictive pericardial disease are likewise excluded from TIPS treatment (Fig 1).

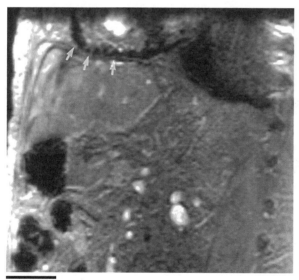

FIGURE 1.
Pericardial calcification. MR venography obtained before transjugular intrahepatic portosystemic shunting to evaluate portal vein patency and hepatic venous anatomy incidentally shows thick, linear area of low signal intensity in the pericardium (*arrows*). This abnormal finding corresponded to a radiodense calcification identified on a lateral chest radiograph, previously misinterpreted as a pleural calcification. The patient was further evaluated and found to have high central venous pressures and cirrhosis secondary to restrictive cardiac disease and was ultimately treated with a pericardiectomy.

Not only would the shunt be ineffective in such patients but also the patient could succumb to right-sided heart failure due to sudden elevation of right atrial pressure. Caution should also be exercised in planning this procedure in patients at risk for atrial arrhythmia or for those in whom such rhythms would be poorly tolerated. For example, in those with known left-bundle branch block, transvenous pacing can be instituted in the same setting as TIPS, as would be required in any manipulation through the right side of the heart in these patients.

A hepatoma, hemangioma, or other neoplasm in the path of the expected tract through the liver contraindicates TIPS. In addition, the procedure should not be performed in the setting of known biliary obstruction, bacterial cholangitis, or acute hepatitis. An active infection, in particular "spontaneous" bacterial peritonitis, should postpone an elective TIPS but will usually not contraindicate an emergent procedure.

Although not commonly encountered, patients with polycystic liver disease were considered to have a contraindication for TIPS because of the risk of bleeding. However, TIPS has been performed in such patients with the assistance of a transfemoral hepatic arterial wire to localize the portal hepatis.

Formerly thought to preclude TIPS, portal venous occlusion is not an absolute contraindication to the procedure. As long as the clot is soft and/or movable, successful performance of TIPS is expected (Fig 2). However, long-standing occlusion associated with cavernous transformation of the portal vein makes conventional TIPS impossible.

Hepatic venous occlusion in Budd-Chiari syndrome can preclude standard TIPS because of the inability to securely access a satisfactory segment of vein from a transjugular approach. However, in some variants of Budd-Chiari, we and others have been successful catheterizing the intrahepatic veins from a percutaneous transhepatic approach and dilating venous webs or stenoses with balloons or recanalizing thrombosed veins. If this is completed before or in conjunction with transjugular catheterization of the veins, TIPS can be performed. In some patients, restoring patency to the central hepatic outflow may obviate the need for portal decompression. Alternately, for patients with hepatic veno-occlusive disease, a direct shunt to the intrahepatic inferior vena cava can be created (Fig 3). In those cases, plans for future liver transplantation need to be considered because the caval stent end may complicate transplant surgery. It should be noted that TIPS does not reduce the intraoperative mortality during liver transplantation and that TIPS is not indicated for transplant "preparation" alone.

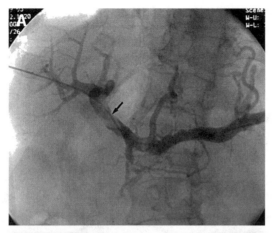

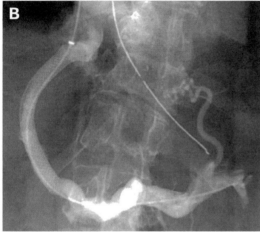

FIGURE 2.
A, portal vein thrombosis. Transhepatic portogram shows partially obstructive filling defects in the portal vein just proximal to the bifurcation, as well as additional defects at the confluence of the superior mesenteric vein and the splenic vein. Coronary and splenic varices are seen. There is no thrombus in the intrahepatic portal venous branches. A transhepatic wire (*arrow*) is left in place as a target for transjugular intrahepatic portosystemic shunting (TIPS) passes. **B,** after TIPS. After TIPS, the thrombus is largely cleared, and there is brisk flow up the stent with minimal intrahepatic portal opacification. Some residual clotting is seen along the stent, and there is still some opacification of varices arising from the splenic vein.

Relative contraindications include renal insufficiency and a history of severe reaction to iodinated contrast. The latter problem can be managed with proper steroid premedication and general anesthesia. The risk of acute tubular necrosis in those with pre-existing renal insufficiency may be acceptable if TIPS is being per-

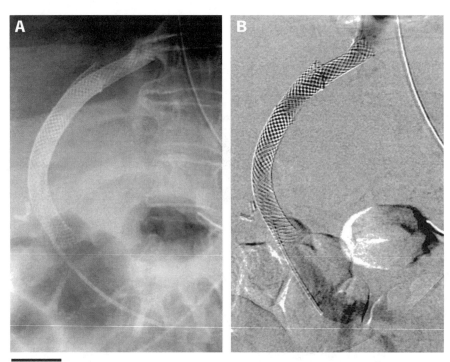

FIGURE 3.
Budd-Chiari stenting to the inferior vena cava. Digital portogram (**A**, unsubtract-ed; **B**, subtracted) using a 5-French multi–sidehole[2AQ] catheter shows three well-expanded, overlapping Wallstents, the most cranial of which extends to the infe-rior vena cava. This positioning was necessary in this patient with Budd-Chiari syndrome and occluded hepatic veins.

formed as a lifesaving measure. In fact, patients with elevated cre-atinine due to hepatorenal syndrome frequently demonstrate improvement in renal function after TIPS.[8,9,12] However, TIPS appears to be less effective at relieving ascites in patients with associated renal insufficiency.[8,13]

Lastly, some centers exclude patients with Child-Pugh scores of greater than 12 as it is generally agreed that the mortality and risk–benefit ratio of the procedure in these patients is unaccept-ably high.

PATIENT PREPARATION BEFORE TRANSJUGULAR INTRAHEPATIC PORTOSYSTEMIC SHUNTING

Before undertaking a TIPS procedure for variceal bleeding, the sur-geon should confirm the variceal source for the bleeding by endo-scopic examination. There are a significant number of patients (15%) who have previously documented variceal bleeding in whom recurrent bleeding is, in fact, not related to varices but to either peptic ulcer disease or Mallory-Weiss tears. Once the variceal source for bleeding is confirmed, unstable patients should be stabilized in an intensive care setting before a TIPS procedure is commenced.

For patients with intractable ascites, it should be confirmed that the ascites is, indeed, intractable and refractive and that management with more conservative measures—diet control, salt restriction, protein restriction, maximal doses of diuretics in suitable patients—has failed.

A detailed history should be obtained from the patient, and in the event that the patient is unable to give consent, a detailed explanation of the procedure with the associated risks, benefits, and expectations should be explained to the family.

Color Doppler US of the liver, portal venous system, and splenic vein should be performed before the TIPS procedure is commenced. This examination should confirm patency of both the hepatic vein and the portal vein, and documentation should also be made of hepatic arterial velocities, the measurement of which would be useful for subsequent follow-up after TIPS placement. A patent splenic vein should be documented, particularly in cases of gastric varices, which may, in fact, be related to splenic vein thrombosis. In such cases, TIPS is not indicated, and a splenectomy is the procedure of choice. In the event that US is unable to confirm the patency of any of the portal vessels or the hepatic vein, MR venography may better evaluate these vessels or further substantiate that these vessels are compromised. An US examination can determine the presence of a hepatoma, polycystic liver disease, and pericardial effusions, any one of which may preclude TIPS and alter patient management.

Significant pulmonary hypertension, right-sided heart failure, and pericardial disease should be ruled out before a TIPS procedure, as the procedure in these situations is associated with a poor outcome.

Preprocedural clinical evaluations should include documentation of a history of encephalopathy and the present degree of encephalopathy, cardiovascular status, the need for a Sengstaken-Blakemore tube if there are actively bleeding varices, the need for airway protection, and paracentesis. Laboratory tests routinely performed before the procedure include a complete blood count, liver function tests, measurement of creatinine concentration, and a coagulation profile, including prothrombin time, international normalized ratio (INR), and partial thromboplastin time. The Child-Pugh score is calculated based on the assessment of encephalopathy, ascites, serum bilirubin concentration, serum albumin concentration, and serum prothrombin time. Prophylactic platelet and/or fresh-frozen plasma transfusions are initiated if the platelet count is less than 30,000 or the INR is greater than 2.0 at the time of the TIPS procedure. A single dose of IV broad-spectrum antibiotics is given before the procedure.

TIPS can be performed with conscious sedation or general anesthesia. General anesthesia offers many advantages, particularly when dealing with an uncooperative patient and in terms of protecting the airway in unconscious patients, providing pain relief, and allowing control of respiration during the technically difficult portion of the examination. However, the procedure can be performed safely with conscious sedation and local anesthesia, provided there is careful patient monitoring by an appropriately trained assistant with knowledge of both conscious sedation and the procedure.

PROCEDURAL TECHNIQUE

For successful TIPS, there is little substitute for experience in performing the procedure. This has been borne out by the fact that there is a lower mortality rate from TIPS at institutions that frequently perform this procedure. During the past 7 years, more than 450 TIPS have been performed at the Beth Israel Deaconess Medical Center. During this period, we have made several modifications to our technique and have learned how to overcome problems posed by small, hard, mobile cirrhotic livers in patients with gross ascites and in situations of difficult hepatic and portal venous anatomy.

Ideally, the right internal jugular vein is used as access to the venous system. However, a right external jugular vein or left internal or external jugular vein can also be used. Although the femoral vein approach has also been reported, we have never had reason to use this access approach.

Early in our experience, we employed the Ring transjugular portal vein access set (Cook, Inc., Bloomington, Ind), which has a modified Colapinto transjugular biopsy needle for puncturing the portal vein through the hepatic vein. The portal vein access needle is a 16G (0.065-inch diameter) reversed beveled hollow needle and is a relatively rigid system. We now prefer the Rosch-Uchida system portal vein access set (Cook, Inc., Bloomington, Ind). This set uses a solid flexible tip 0.038-inch diameter pointed needle, advanced within a 5.2-French (F) (0.068-inch diameter) straight catheter to gain access to the portal vein. We believe this produces a less traumatic puncture than an angled cutting needle configuration.

More recently, a fine needle (21G; 0.032-inch diameter) has been used to cannulate the portal vein with the assistance of CO_2 and a 0.018-inch wire. Advocates maintain that this is a safer, less traumatic access system. No benefit has been demonstrated in the literature between this fine-needle system and the other larger systems.

Preferably, the right hepatic vein is cannulated with a 5-F catheter and the assistance of a 0.035-inch guide wire. Once the hepatic vein is cannulated, a contrast venogram should be performed to ensure that there is no central hepatic venous stenosis. This can predispose the shunt to intimal hyperplasia and subsequent shunt failure. After the catheter and wire system are advanced into the right hepatic vein (usually the easiest to cannulate), the sheath is advanced over the catheter wire system so that the tip of the sheath is well within the hepatic vein. Next, a balloon occlusion catheter is positioned through the sheath and into the hepatic vein for hepatic wedge venography and portal vein localization. Although this balloon occlusion catheter can be advanced over 0.025-inch wire, the balloon catheter alone can usually easily be passed through the sheath after the 5-F catheter and 0.035-inch wire have been removed. Care should be taken to ensure that the thin-walled 10-F sheath does not kink with respiratory motion, as this can cause difficulty with advancing of the portal venous access system later in the procedure.

Some method of portal vein localization has always been performed during the TIPS procedure in our institution. However, some investigators do not perform this at all before going on to the next stage of the procedure, which is the attempted puncture between the hepatic vein and the portal venous system. Multiple techniques of real-time and non–real-time portal vein localization have been described. Non–real-time techniques include hepatic wedge venography with iodinated contrast and carbon dioxide (CO_2) and late-phase superior mesenteric arteriography. Real-time methods include US-guided percutaneous placement of microcoils adjacent to the portal vein, real-time color Doppler US-guided puncture of the portal vein from the hepatic vein, umbilical vein catheterization, placement of radiopaque wire in the hepatic artery, and US-guided percutaneous placement of a 0.018-inch wire into the portal vein.

We now almost exclusively use hepatic wedge portography with CO_2 for portal vein localization before portal venous access. For the CO_2 wedge portogram, 50 cc of CO_2 is injected by hand injection in a rapid fashion, using a digital subtraction technique with at least two frames per second. Using this technique, both the intrahepatic and extrahepatic portal venous structures are opacified in greater than 90% of cases (Fig 4). Preferentially, the more nondependent intrahepatic and portal venous structures are opacified with CO_2, which does not pose any problems and does not detract from the usefulness of this technique. CO_2 portography has

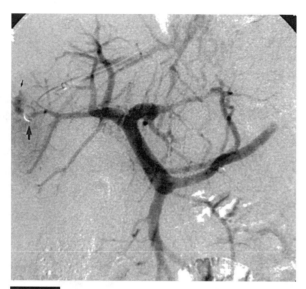

FIGURE 4.

Digital subtraction hepatic wedge portography with CO_2. After catheterization of the right hepatic vein and advancement of a 10-French transjugular intrahepatic portosystemic shunt sheath, a balloon occlusion catheter is used to obtain a wedged CO_2 venogram (*large arrow*, balloon inflated on balloon occlusion catheter; *tiny arrow*, parenchymal stain from wedged test injection). Both frontal and lateral projections are obtained, and clear images of the portal circulation are consistently achieved.

the advantage of not contributing toward iodinated contrast burden. Although we had one case of capsule perforation related to the wedge CO_2 injection, this occurred without consequence, and we have had no clinically significant complication related to the use of CO_2.

Separate wedge venograms are performed in both the anteroposterior and lateral positions (obviously, if biplane facilities are available, a single injection will do). With CO_2, the more nondependent portal radicals are especially well seen, and this can include the recanalized umbilical vein. We believe that imaging in the lateral plane is especially important to verify whether the catheter is positioned in the right hepatic vein or the middle hepatic vein. Anteroposterior imaging alone cannot always differentiate this. Obviously, this has important consequences, as an anterior puncture from the middle hepatic vein will result in an extracapsular puncture. Catheter position may be indicated by the arrow on the Rosch-Uschida cannula: if it points more posteriorly, the cannula is in the right hepatic vein, whereas if the arrow points more anterolaterally, it is in the middle hepatic vein. The antero-posterior projection is used to determine the bone landmarks of the portal vein. Obviously, however, these change with respiration, and, in fact, when the cannula system is rotated during the attempted portal venous puncture, the liver itself may move, which makes these bone references only rough guides as to the level of the portal vein. Indeed, the liver movement in patients with gross ascites, particularly when the liver is small, may be as much as 5 to 6 cm. This movement may be in not only the mediolateral plane but also the cephalocaudad axis. For localizing the portal system in such a mobile liver, real-time localization is beneficial, and for this, we have used US-guided percutaneous transhepatic placement of a 0.018-inch wire into the portal vein successfully.

CO_2-wedged venography gives an estimate as to how far the needle can be advanced without extracapsular puncture. However, this technique is not a real-time method of localizing the portal vein, and thus, extracapsular puncture cannot always be avoided. We have had extracapsular punctures in 15 of our last 100 cases using this technique. The reported rates for this have been as high as 50% in the literature. Since we have started using the Rosch-Uchida set, these extracapsular punctures have not been associated with any significant bleeding episodes.

When puncturing from the hepatic vein to the portal vein, we usually attempt to exit the hepatic vein in its proximal portion within 3 to 4 cm of the inferior vena cava. By doing this, needle passes caudad to the target portal vein can be avoided. Also, acutely angled (kinked) shunts between the more peripheral portal and hepatic venous branches can result from the distal hepatic vein exit site. The portal vein is ideally entered within 3 cm of the bifurcation. However, entry too close to the bifurcation risks extrahepatic puncture of the portal vein. The portal bifurcation has been demonstrated to be extrahepatic in 48% of cases and at the liver capsule in 25% of cases.

For portal vein cannulation, the metal cannula is rotated appropriately, the portal vein puncturing system is advanced, and a contrast-filled syringe is initially aspirated until blood return is achieved. Contrast injection confirms the portal vein cannulations. Then, a guide wire is advanced into the main portal vein and either the superior mesenteric vein or the splenic vein. Subsequently, a 5-F multi–sidehole catheter is advanced into the main portal vein for portography and pressure measurements. Pitfalls at this stage of the procedure include cannulation of the hepatic artery or bile ducts. These should be recognized if an appropriate technique has been used.

After portography and pressure measurements are performed, the parenchymal tract can be dilated. (If there is any question of an extrahepatic portal venous puncture, this access should be abandoned.) For dilation of the parenchymal tract, usually a 10-mm balloon catheter is used. However, in hard, cirrhotic livers, predilation with a smaller 4 to 6mm balloon catheter may be needed, or, in more difficult cases, a Van Andel catheter (Cook, Bloomington, Ind) can be used. Predilation can also be achieved using the Rosch-Uchida set by advancing the 10-F polytetrafluoroethylene catheter over the catheter–wire combination.

Once a stiff multipurpose wire (0.035-inch × 180-cm Amplatz superstiff guide wire; Meditech, Watertown, Mass) has secured the portal venous access, the Rosch-Uchida portal vein access set can be removed. Parenchymal dilation is performed before placement of the stent. Before stent deployment, careful consideration is given to anatomical landmarks, such as the hepatocaval junction and the relations of the venous tract to portal venous structures. The shunt should not extend into the inferior vena cava or within 3 cm of the splenomesenteric vein confluence if future technically complicated transplantation is to be avoided (Fig 5). Although many different stents have been used for TIPS, most institutions in the United States use the Wallstent (Schneider [USA] Inc., Pfizer Technology Group, Minneapolis, Minn) (Fig 6). At least a 1-cm length of stent should extend beyond both the hepatic venous and portal venous ends of the parenchymal tract, as continued shortening after deployment can be expected.

Although we predominantly use 10-mm diameter stents, there may be situations, specifically, marked hepatofugal flow, very large varices, and dramatically elevated portosystemic gradients (greater than 30 mm Hg), in which a 12-mm stent may be preferable. In this situation, a 12-mm stent can be dilated up to 10 mm initially, and the subsequent portosystemic gradient can then be evaluated to determine whether dilation to 12 mm is necessary. Excessive shunting causes encephalopathy. Rarely, the portosystemic gradient remains above 12 mm Hg after placement of a 10-mm stent and dilation to 10 mm. Overdilation of a 10-mm stent to 12 mm can be performed but may result in serious distortion of the stent. Although it has been described that parallel stents may be required to adequately reduce portosystemic gradients in some cases, we have never had to do this in our experience of more than 450 TIPS procedures.

Immediately after the transjugular intrahepatic portosystemic shunt is positioned, repeat portosystemic pressure measurements should be obtained, confirming that the pressure gradient is below 12 mm Hg. Invariably, a rise in the central venous pressure is

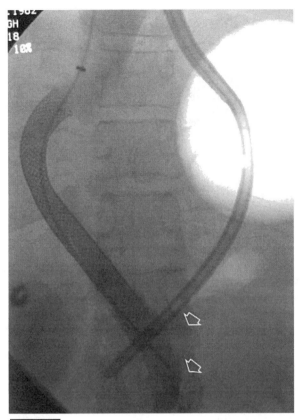

FIGURE 5.
Importance of stent positioning relative to splenomesenteric vein confluence. Portogram after emergent transjugular intrahepatic portosystemic
shunting shows the stent extending far into the portal vein (*arrows* indicate orifices of splenic and superior mesenteric veins). Note the inflated
Sengstaken-Blakemore tube. Had this patient been a candidate for liver
transplantation, the stent in this location would likely interfere with
surgery.

noted at this time, and for patients with pericardial effusions, very
close monitoring is necessary.

The decision to embolize varices during TIPS remains a controversial topic. It is recognized that, despite having the portosystemic gradient reduced to below 12 mm Hg, a number of patients
can still continue to bleed. The reason for this continued bleeding
despite adequate portal decompression remains unclear. It may be
related to severe coagulopathy. Consequently, it is our policy in
patients who have had life-threatening variceal bleeding and severe
coagulopathy (INR > 1.8 and platelet count < 50,000) to perform
variceal embolization at the time of the TIPS procedure. A possible

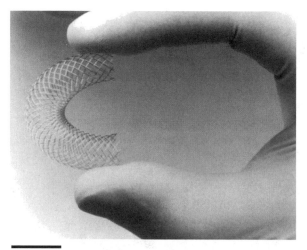

FIGURE 6.
Wallstent endoprosthesis (Schneider [USA] Inc., Pfizer Technology Group; Minneapolis, Minn). Note the flexibility of this unconstrained stainless steel metal mesh stent, which also has radial force. (Courtesy of Boston Scientific/Vascular, Natick, Mass.)

added benefit of this is increasing hepatopetal flow, which may improve hepatocyte perfusion as well as shunt patency. Variceal embolization can be achieved with a variety of embolic materials, which include absolute ethanol, gelfoam (Upjohn Company, Kalamazoo, Mich) or coils.

Although portal venous thrombosis is considered to be a relative contraindication to TIPS, TIPS has been successfully performed in this situation. An initial transhepatic approach can be used to localize the portal vein, but we have found that conventional transjugular approach allows transjugular intrahepatic portosystemic shunt formation in these cases. It is not desirable nor has it been necessary to use thrombolytic therapy to recanalize the portal veins; mechanical thrombectomy is the preferred method. This can be achieved by either suction thrombectomy, balloon insertion, or more sophisticated mechanical thrombectomy devices.[14]

POSTPROCEDURAL CARE

All patients spend the first day and night after TIPS in an ICU, and bed rest is ordered. The indwelling 10-F TIPS sheath is exchanged for a short 7- to 8-F central venous catheter. If obtaining jugular venous access was difficult or if central venous pressure measurements are required, there may be some advantage to maintaining internal jugular access (e.g., if the need for immediate reintervention arises). Vital signs are closely monitored, and the jugular venous access site is evaluated for the presence of a hematoma, bleeding, or both. Most patients do best with the head of the bed elevated, and many require a small pressure dressing, which is anticipated in this population with coagulopathies.

Complaints of abdominal pain are worrisome; in general, the jugular venous access site should be the only sore area after the procedure has been performed. Pain medications should not be necessary in most patients. Complications that may present with abdominal signs or symptoms include intraparenchymal or intraperitoneal hemorrhages or bile peritonitis, the latter being very rare. Intraperitoneal bleeding is the most feared early complication and is monitored by measurement of serial hematocrit levels, physical examination, and charting heart rate and blood pressure. Hematocrit levels are measured every 6 to 8 hours overnight. In evaluating vital signs, it should be noted that functioning shunt releases gut-derived vasoactive substances directly into the systemic circulation, which results in diminished peripheral arterial resistance (expected) and, thus, mild arterial hypotension.[15]

At many centers, TIPS is performed with local anesthesia and conscious sedation alone. At our institution, first-time TIPS procedures are invariably performed under general anesthesia. Patients can usually be extubated at the end of the procedure while still in the angiography suite. However, a minority of patients will have extubation delayed or will require supplemental oxygen. As soon as the patient can be placed upright, an upright chest radiograph is obtained to exclude any pneumothorax related to jugular venous punctures and also to evaluate heart size and pulmonary vasculature after shunt formation. High output heart failure is very unlikely if patients are screened for cardiac abnormalities before TIPS, but an increase in cardiac index and a corresponding decrease in peripheral and pulmonary vascular resistance should be anticipated.[15]

All patients have at least one large-bore peripheral IV line that should be maintained for rapid fluid resuscitation or transfusion of blood products, if necessary. Gentle parenteral hydration is continued at least overnight, especially if patients still cannot tolerate oral fluids. Five percent dextrose in water can be used for patients with sodium restrictions (those with ascites and/or hydrothorax). The urinary catheter placed for the procedure is also maintained for accurate determination of fluid balance. This is especially important for patients at risk for acute tubular necrosis, that is, those with preexisting renal insufficiency, those who received large contrast loads, or those who experienced prolonged hypotension. Serum creatinine levels are monitored while patients are hospitalized.

Emergent TIPS procedures may need to be performed with an inflated Sengstaken-Blakemore tube in place. With satisfactory reduction in portal venous pressure after TIPS, the tube balloon can be deflated. After TIPS, a portal angiogram taken with the balloon deflated is reassuring evidence of successful decompression of varices. In most cases, the esophageal tube itself is left in position overnight but is deflated.

This same subset of patients treated emergently may be receiving IV octreotide to decrease splanchnic blood flow. The drug should be discontinued after transjugular intrahepatic portosystemic shunt placement because the diminished portal flow may potentially result in early stent occlusion. This is of particular concern in patients with relatively normal coagulation parameters (Fig 7). For this reason, we administer prophylactic heparin to these TIPS patients overnight (a very small subset of all patients), provided there were no extracapsular hepatic punctures during the procedure.

The patient care team needs to anticipate possible new or worsened hepatic encephalopathy after portosystemic shunting. In the majority of cases, this is medically controllable with lactulose, neomycin, and protein restriction. New onset encephalopathy or

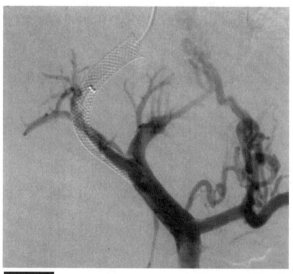

FIGURE 7.
Early thrombosis after transjugular intrahepatic portosystemic shunting (TIPS). Less than 24 hours after successful TIPS, this patient with a relatively normal coagulation status returned for reintervention when an US examination showed the absence of blood flow in the stent. Contrast portography shows opacification of intrahepatic portal venous branches and previously decompressed varices. The fully expanded, well-positioned stent is completely occluded. This soft, new thrombus was easily cleared with a balloon, and no additional stenting was required. The patient received anticoagulation for 48 hours after this revision.

severe encephalopathy should, however, raise the concern of possible hepatic failure. Thus, the clinical picture needs to be evaluated in conjunction with laboratory and other data. Liver function tests are reviewed on a daily basis while patients are hospitalized. Rarely, incapacitating encephalopathy will require reintervention to reduce the shunt with a reducing stent or stent occlusion.

A baseline sonographic examination of the new transjugular intrahepatic portosystemic shunt is obtained the day after the procedure, as will be discussed in the Surveillance section. Detection of abnormal flow patterns suggesting significant stenosis or occlusion requires prompt intervention and possible revision.

RESULTS

The technical success of TIPS is now in excess of 93%, and procedure-related mortality rates range between 1% and 3%. For patients with variceal bleeding and ascites, initial clinical success can be achieved in 85% to 95% of patients.[8,12,16,17]

Cumulative survival rates at 30 days range between 85% and 97%. Acute Physiology and Chronic Health Evaluation scores greater than 18 and co-morbidities are directly related to mortality after TIPS procedures. Multiorgan failure and liver failure are the most common causes of death within 30 days of TIPS procedures. Cumulative long-term survival rates after TIPS are 85% at 30 days, 70% at 1 year, and 56% at 2 years. On the basis of Child-Pugh class classification, cumulative survival rates at 2 years are 75% for Child-Pugh class A, 55% for class B, and 43% for class C.[18,19]

Recurrent upper gastrointestinal bleeding can be expected in 15% to 30% of patients. Approximately 15% to 20% of these cases, however, are secondary to nonvariceal causes, such as Mallory-Weiss tears or peptic ulcer disease.

TIPS procedures have been shown to be of clinical benefit in more than 75% of patients in whom TIPS was performed for intractable ascites. Patients in whom TIPS is performed for variceal bleeding have also demonstrated a dramatic improvement in ascites after the procedure. The absence of preprocedural renal insufficiency is the only characteristic identified as an indicator of clinical success for TIPS in intractable ascites. Independent risk factors for poor outcomes after TIPS for patients with intractable ascites include persistent alcohol use and elevated creatinine and elevated total bilirubin levels. Therefore, careful consideration should be given to these factors before any proposed TIPS procedure in these patients.

COMPLICATIONS[12,16,19,20]

Complications of TIPS can be arbitrarily divided into those specific to the procedure itself, particularly the transparenchymal puncture, those associated with creation of the portosystemic shunt with a stent, and those known to be associated with any invasive, angiographic study using iodinated contrast.

The most dreaded complication, specific to the relatively blind hepatic puncture, is transcapsular instrument passage resulting in life-threatening intraperitoneal hemorrhaging. In reality, capsular transgression alone, without an associated vascular puncture, is usually without clinically apparent consequence. Nevertheless, it is helpful to be aware that such an injury has occurred, and we routinely inject a tiny amount of contrast at each needle pass, before aspirating for portal venous blood, to see whether the capsule has been violated. If the more traumatic Colapinto system is used, it may be prudent to embolize such a tract, and this should definitely be performed if the transcapsular pass also punctures a blood vessel. In the worst scenario, the portal vein itself may be accessed in a central, extrahepatic location, unbeknownst to the operators, who dilate the portal vein at an extrahepatic site using a balloon catheter, essentially rupturing the portal vein. Catastrophic exsanguination can result, and this has been described in the literature. Although a covered stent may prove to be valuable in this situation, placement of an uncovered stent can prevent significant hemorrhaging and the need for surgical intervention. An arterial puncture, even without any associated capsular injury, can result in an intraparenchymal or subcapsular hematoma. Again, direct tract embolization is probably the best option for immediate treatment (if the punctured branch is large) because transfemoral intraluminal arterial embolization would put the patient at high risk for liver failure or an infarct after TIPS. Superselective arterial branch embolization, however, might be tolerated. An extraparenchymal hepatic arterial puncture at the porta is potentially more disastrous, resulting in perihepatic hemorrhaging. Immediate percutaneous treatment in such a situation would involve transfemoral access for complete transluminal arterial embolization (precluding TIPS or putting the patient at severe risk for hepatic failure after TIPS) or open surgical repair.

The biliary tree is subject to traversal during TIPS, and transient, self-limited hemobilia is reported to occur in 1% to 4% of cases. Biliary obstruction can occur after TIPS. More worrisome is creation of the shunt across a bile duct, resulting in a biliary-venous fistula. In the short term, an elevated serum bilirubin level, hemobilia, and (possibly) sepsis, may result. More importantly, in the long term, this transgression is strongly associated with accelerated neointimal hyperplasia within the stent and recurrent stent occlusion (Fig 8).[21,22] To avoid this, some investigators advocate an "over-the-wire" contrast study of the TIPS tract before balloon dilation: if a bile duct is opacified, the access is aborted and a new puncture is made.

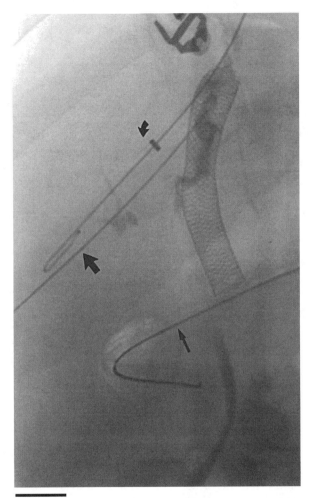

FIGURE 8.
Occluded stent related to a biliary-venous fistula. Reintervention for
occluded transjugular intrahepatic portosystemic shunt stent: CO_2 portography had demonstrated complete occlusion of the stent with a patent
portal system. Attempts at catheterizing this occluded stent from the
transjugular route were unsuccessful, which prompted direct transhepatic puncture of the stent with a 21-gauge needle (*thick black arrow*). With
the needle tip in the stent, contrast injection demonstrates bile duct opacification, indicating a biliary fistula, which is the likely reason for the
occlusion. *Narrow arrow*, distal end of the nasogastric tube; *curved arrow*,
10-French sheath and J-wire in hepatic vein.

Alternatively, if discovered after stent deployment, the communication can be closed off by placement of a covered stent.

During attempts to access the hepatic veins, aggressive
catheter and guide wire manipulations can trigger atrial arrhyth-

mia or, worse, can lacerate the relatively thin right ventricle. Although we have not experienced the latter type of cardiac complication in a first-time TIPS procedure, one difficult TIPS revision was complicated by the puncture of the right ventricle, with resultant intrapericardial hemorrhaging and tamponade, requiring emergent decompression. This patient eventually underwent successful TIPS recanalization. Transient arrhythmias are reported to occur in less than 5% of procedures,[20] although Pidlich et al.[23] monitored 12 patents before, during, and after TIPS and detected supraventricular and ventricular tachyarrhythmia in 9 of the 12 patients. We have had one patient in the past 8 years who had a persistent but hemodynamically stable atrial tachycardia that required medical therapy during the intervention but that resolved after the procedure, without sequelae.

Aberrant punctures may also potentially injure the right kidney or adrenal gland or the colon, but these complications are extremely rare and should not occur when the procedure is performed by an experienced interventionalist.

Complications related to the portosystemic shunt itself can be divided into physiologic and metal-stent–related complications. As previously described, a successful shunt causes a relatively sudden increase in venous blood return to the right atrium, which, in susceptible patients, can result in acute congestive heart failure and pulmonary edema. Careful patient selection and judicious hydration should make this a very unusual occurrence.

The diversion of high-pressure portal venous blood away from bleeding varices necessarily shunts the blood from the liver as well. Many patients with cirrhosis show an "arterialized" hepatic blood supply and tolerate the procedure's shunting of portal flow because of a relative compensatory increase in hepatic arterial flow. In those with less arterial compensation, there is a risk of progressive liver dysfunction and, ultimately, liver failure after TIPS. Approximately 10% to 20% of patients show a transient elevation in the levels of their liver function tests after shunting, which peaks during the week after the procedure; acute, massive hepatic failure probably occurs in less than 5% of patients. These results are not dissimilar from liver failure rates after nonselective surgical shunts.[24,25]

Diversion of portal venous blood also accounts for one of the more common and frustrating complications of TIPS, that is, new or worsened hepatic encephalopathy, occurring in 15% to 35% of patients after TIPS. This rate is greater than might be expected for creation of similar-sized nonselective surgical shunts. The reason for the discrepancy is unclear. Factors associated with an increased likelihood of significant encephalopathy after TIPS, other than a previous history of encephalopathy, include age older than 60 years, severe liver impairment (patients with Child-Pugh's class C status), and non–alcoholic-related liver disease. Creation of a larger diameter shunt (12 mm vs. 8-10 mm) also appears to result in more encephalopathy. Fortunately, this is medically controllable in the majority of those affected, but approximately 5% remain persistently disabled. As stated previously, severe encephalopathy can necessitate intentional reduction or occlusion of the transjugular intrahepatic portosystemic shunt. Several techniques have been devised for reducing stents,[26] one of which is a stenotic stent, which may be produced or constructed by tying a constraining 3-0 suture around the midportion of a partially deployed, reconstrainable Wallstent (Schneider [USA] Inc.). These reducing stents provide a measure of continued portal system decompression while relieving encephalopathy related to excessive shunting. If this reducing stent is not effective, however, there may be a rare occasion when total occlusion of the shunt is required.

Placement of a stent within the vascular system always carries some risk of malposition or migration of the device. Freedman et al.[20] reported a 1% to 3% malposition or migration rate from a review of 20 sources reported up to 1993. We have had no difficulties with stability of the Wallstent endoprosthesis (Schneider [USA] Inc.) for TIPS. Because the Wallstent is flexible, capable of being reconstrained, and self-expanding, it is popular for use in TIPS; however, because of shortening of the Wallstent with expansion, its final position is less predictable, before deployment, than is that of other commonly used stents. This may result in improper or imprecise stent positioning. During and after deployment, contrast injection, "road-mapping" techniques, and additional oblique views can assist the operator in determining where the stent will finally reside in relation to the hepatic and portal venous margins. Adequate balloon dilation of the tract before stenting, recognition of plans for future transplantation, and, importantly, experience should minimize deployment and positioning problems. Successful percutaneous retrieval of misplaced stents has been described by several authors.[27]

Another complication associated with the presence of the stent within the vascular system is a transient hemolytic syndrome. Invariably self-limited, this is usually detected by a decrease in the hemoglobin level and usually subsides in 3 to 4 months without treatment.[28]

Although the portal vein is capable of withstanding considerable manipulation as part of the TIPS procedure, there is a potential for venous dissection or other injuries, particularly in those who have hypoalbuminemia. This is rare. Less unusual is portal venous thrombosis after TIPS, which may progress because of prolonged intervention, a pre-existing clot, the presence of the stent end in the vein, and competitive shunts decreasing hepatopetal flow. If we cannot, using angiography, confirm brisk hepatopetal flow through a fully expanded stent after the procedure (even with an acceptable gradient), we will embolize large gastroesophageal and splenic varices competing for portal venous outflow. We are more wary of therapeutic embolization of spontaneous splenorenal, mesocaval, or mesoiliac shunts.

Acute occlusion of the TIPS stent may occur with or without associated portal venous thrombosis. In our experience, predisposing factors include normal coagulation parameters, insufficient stent length or stent shortening, extreme shunt angulation or tortuosity, and poor inflow, the latter usually being secondary to large competitive spontaneous shunts with hepatofugal or to-and-fro sluggish portal blood flow. Intraprocedural embolization of varices and postprocedural anticoagulation in select patients are measures taken to avoid this complication. Self-expanding stents may gradually shorten after the procedure, which results in displacement of a stent end out of the vein and into the parenchymal tract, which is another cause of occlusion. For this latter reason, we fully expand stents using a balloon catheter during placement to determine the final length and position, and we always position the stent well into the hepatic venous lumen. Noninvasive shunt interrogation should be performed within 24 hours of TIPS to detect these early failures so that recanalization can be performed expediently. Early revisions may simply entail suction or mechanical thrombectomy of a fresh, soft clot but may also require further stent dilatation, stent extension, or variceal embolization.

Delayed stenosis of the hepatic vein just beyond the hepatic venous end of the TIPS stent is a frequent problem. Extension of a length of metal stent into the hepatic vein, sometimes nearly to its origin, is important in reducing hepatic venous end stenosis after TIPS. However, delayed shunt stenosis and occlusion related to intimal hyperplasia either within or at the hepatic venous end of the stent remain the Achilles' heel of TIPS. The eventual occurrence of such narrowing is one of the reasons that regular clinical and sonographic shunt follow-up is so important.

Infectious complications may be associated with even minimally invasive procedures. Although unusual in our experience, sepsis has been reported by some centers to occur in up to 10% of patients.[20] As previously described, we routinely administer prophylactic IV antibiotics before TIPS.

Risks related to jugular venous punctures include hematomas, carotid artery punctures, arteriovenous fistulas, hemothorax, and pneumothorax. When complicated jugular venous access is anticipated, sonographic guidance should be used. After the procedure, we obtain an upright chest radiograph to determine whether thoracic complications are present. In addition, during dilatation of the tract to the vein for passage of the large TIPS sheath and during subsequent manipulations, one must also keep in mind possible inadvertent carotid "massage," inducing bradycardia.

The administration of iodinated contrast material always carries a risk of inducing nausea and vomiting and idiosyncratic reactions such as rashes, cardiac arrhythmia, hypotension, or, most disturbingly, acute laryngospasm or sudden death. We perform all TIPS under general anesthesia, and our patients have not experienced these particular contrast-related complications. However, careful preangiographic historical screening to identify patients who warrant use of nonionic contrast material and steroid premedication should prevent many of these reactions. Many centers have abandoned use of regular ionic contrast.

Acute renal failure from acute tubular necrosis is another well-known untoward effect of iodinated contrast, particularly for those individuals with already compromised renal function. Although adequate preprocedural hydration is the single best preventive step for avoiding this complication, TIPS is often performed on an emergent basis, which limits hydration, and, indeed, in many patients with cirrhosis, it may be difficult to optimize intravascular volume without increasing ascites and edema. Use of digital subtraction technology allows lower concentrations and volumes of contrast to be used while preserving image quality, and use of CO_2 as a contrast agent can further decrease the total iodinated contrast load. Fortunately, in our experience and that of others, TIPS-associated renal failure is unusual, occurring in less than 1% to 4% of cases.

As with any complex, invasive procedure, a small but real risk of a periprocedural myocardial infarction or stroke exists. Therefore, intraprocedural oximetry and hemodynamic monitoring are mandatory, whether conscious sedation or general anesthesia is used.

The relatively prolonged fluoroscopy times over a small area during TIPS procedures has, in isolated cases, resulted in radiation-induced skin changes. Erythema and hair loss has been described, occurring on the backs of patients in a distribution corresponding to the imaging field of view used during TIPS. Tertiary centers, treating a patient after one or more unsuccessful attempts at TIPS elsewhere, need to be especially aware of the patient's cumulative dose and should angle the fluoroscopic tube accordingly to avoid irradiating the same area of skin. Radiation exposure is a risk for both the patient and the operator. As this and other complex interventions using ionizing radiation for imaging proliferate, judicious coning, shielding, and tube angulation should be used, and limits of exposure and the procedure duration must be carefully considered.

TRANSJUGULAR INTRAHEPATIC PORTOSYSTEMIC SHUNTING PATENCY AND SURVEILLANCE

Although TIPS has short-term efficacy at reducing portal pressure and stopping variceal hemorrhaging, the ultimate sucess of TIPS depends on its long-term efficacy in preventing recurrent bleeding, in relieving ascites, and in maintaining a reduction in portal pressure. The major limitation on the long-term efficacy of TIPS is shunt patency. Stenosis or occlusion of the transjugular intrahepatic portosystemic shunt with recurrence of portal hypertension has been reported in 17% to 50% of patients at 6 months after TIPS insertion and in 23% to 87% at 12 months.[12,16,19,29,30] With interventions, primary-assisted and secondary patency rates can be 83% and 79%, respectively, at 1 year and 96% and 90%, respectively, at 2 years.[31]

Transjugular intrahepatic portosystemic shunt stenosis and occlusion are caused by three basic mechanisms: (1) acute thrombosis within 30 days, which is usually related to mechanical kinking or shortening of the stent (Fig 9), (2) pseudointimal hyperplasia within the stent and parenchymal tract, which is associated with underlying biliary fistulas, and (3) intimal hyperplasia within the outflow hepatic vein. Acute thrombosis may rarely occur without a mechanical cause in a group of patients with relatively normal platelet counts and INRs less than 1.5. These patients may benefit from postprocedure anticoagulation, provided that there were no intraprocedural extracapsular hepatic punctures. Parenchymal tract stenoses and occlusions are the major cause of symptomatic shunt failure after transjugular intrahepatic portosystemic shunt formation. Although common, hepatic vein stenoses are infrequently associated with recurrent symptoms.[21]

Color Doppler US is the least invasive method of TIPS surveillance and is extremely accurate in detecting shunt occlusion.[32-34] However, it appears to be less accurate in predicting transjugular intrahepatic portosystemic shunt stenosis associated with significant portal hypertension. The occurrence and degree of stenosis is best documented by portal venography along with measurements of portal pressures. Detailed US examination of intrastent, portal venous, and hepatic arterial flow

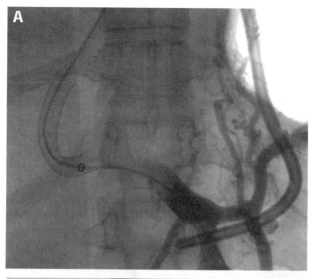

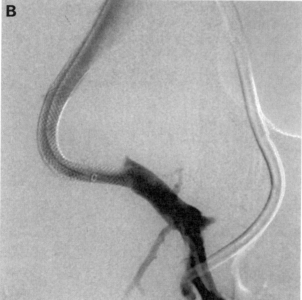

FIGURE 9.
Early transjugular intrahepatic portosystemic shunting (TIPS) and portal vein thrombosis. **A,** portogram taken at the time of TIPS revision shows no opacification of the distal portal vein or stent. Varices are filling despite the presence of an inflated gastroesophageal balloon tube. The findings corresponded to US diagnosis of shunt thrombosis. Catheter suction thrombectomy and mechanical clot maceration with a balloon failed to restore adequate shunt patency, probably because of stent angulation (kink). **B,** consequently, a further buttressing stent was placed coaxially with a good effect.

parameters with comparison to baseline US examinations after TIPS can also predict significant stenosis. In many centers, surveillance is currently performed using color Doppler US every 3 months for the first year and every 6 months thereafter.

FUTURE

Currently, one of the vexing problems with TIPS is the unpredictable but nearly inevitable occurrence of shunt stenosis, as already described. Secondary to a combination of exuberant intimal hyperplasia within the stent and in the stented vein, the narrowing can progress to eventual occlusion, often from superimposed thrombosis.[35] One percutaneous remedy presently available is the use of stent grafts (covered stents) for the shunt. Manufactured with a polytetrafluoroethylene or polyester sleeve over a stainless steel flexible metal mesh stent, these can also be hand fashioned in the angiography suite. Animal studies have clearly demonstrated improved shunt patency when covered stents are used in TIPS.[36] Most human data available as of this writing refer to use of stent grafts placed at the time of a TIPS revision,[37] but investigators are using covered stents for first-time TIPS with definite benefits in terms of shunt patency. As has already been mentioned, covered stents are also important in the percutaneous treatment of TIPS complications such as a biliary-venous fistula or an extracapsular portal venous entrance. More work is needed to assess the best graft materials, stent types, and delivery devices for this promising improvement to TIPS. In addition, adjuvant therapies, such as local irradiation, or drug delivery may prove to be effective in diminishing obstructive neointimal hyperplasia. The role of anticoagulation and antiplatelet agents in promoting TIPS patency has yet to be defined.

In addition, progress in preprocedural physiologic evaluation may more accurately predict a susceptibility to acute hepatic failure, cardiac decompensation, and encephalopathy, which would result in better patient selection.

Although simultaneous advances in other medical and surgical therapies may delay or even eliminate the need for TIPS in some patients, this procedure presently holds an important place in treating complications of portal hypertension.

REFERENCES

1. Gusberg RJ: Distal splenorenal shunt: Premise, perspective, practice. *Dig Dis* 10:84S-93S, 1992.
2. Colapinto RF, Stronell RD, Birch SJ, et al: Creation of an intrahepatic portosystemic shunt with a Gruntzig balloon catheter. *CMAJ* 126:267-268, 1982.

3. Rosch J, Hanafee WN, Snow H: Transjugular portal venography and radiologic portacaval shunt: An experimental study. *Radiology* 92:1112-1114, 1969.

4. Palmaz JC, Sibbitt RR, Reuter SR, et al: Expandable intrahepatic portacaval shunt stents: Early experience in the dog. *AJR Am J Roentgenol* 145:821-825, 1985.

5. Rosch J, Uchida BT, Putnam JS, et al: Experimental intrahepatic portacaval anastomosis: Use of expandable Gianturco stents. *Radiology* 162:481-485, 1987.

6. Richter GM, Palmaz JC, Noeldge G, et al: The transjugular intrahepatic portosystemic stent-shunt (TIPSS). A new nonsurgical percutaneous method. *Radiology* 29:406-411, 1989.

7. Richter GM, Noeldge G, Palmaz JC, et al: The transjugular intrahepatic portosystemic stent-shunt (TIPSS): Results of a pilot study. *Cardiovasc Intervent Radiol* 13:200-207, 1990.

8. Crenshaw WB, Gordon FD, McEniff NJ, et al: Severe ascites: Efficacy of the transjugular intrahepatic portosystemic shunt in treatment. *Radiology* 200:185-192, 1996.

9. Martinet JP, Fenyves D, Legault L, et al: Treatment of refractory ascites using transjugular intrahepatic portosystemic shunt (TIPS): A caution. *Dig Dis Sci* 42:161-166, 1997.

10. Sellinger M, Ochs A, Haag K, et al: Incidence of hepatic encephalopathy and follow-up of liver function in patients with TIPS. *Gastroenterology* 62:883A, 1992.

11. Sahugun G, Brenner KG, Barton RE, et al: Encephalopathy, ascites and hepatic synthetic function after TIPS for variceal hemorrhage. *Hepatology* 16:80A, 1992.

12. LaBerge JM, Ring EJ, Gordon RL, et al: Creation of transjugular intrahepatic portosystemic shunts with the Wallstent endoprosthesis: Results in 100 patients. *Radiology* 187:413-420, 1993.

13. Nazarian GK, Bjarnason H, Dietz CA Jr, et al: Refractory ascites: Midterm results of treatment with a transjugular intrahepatic portosystemic shunt. *Radiology* 205:173-180, 1997.

14. Radosevich PM, Ring EJ, LaBerge JM, et al: Transjugular intrahepatic portosystemic shunts in patients with portal vein occlusion. *Radiology* 186:523-527, 1993.

15. Colombato LA, Spahr L, Martinet J-P, et al: Haemodynamic adaptation two months after transjugular intrahepatic portosystemic shunt (TIPS) in cirrhotic patients. *Gut* 39:600-604, 1996.

16. Rössle M, Haag K, Ochs A, et al: The transjugular intrahepatic portosystemic stent-shunts for variceal bleeding. *N Engl J Med* 330:165-171, 1994.

17. Saxon RR, Keller FS: Technical aspects of accessing the portal vein during the TIPS procedure. *J Vasc Interv Radiol* 8:733-744, 1997.

18. Rubin RA, Haskal ZJ, O'Brien CB, et al: Transjugular intrahepatic portosystemic shunting: Decreased survival for patients with high APACHE II scores. *Am J Gastroenterol* 90:556-563, 1995.

19. Coldwell DM, Ring EJ, Rees CR, et al: Multicenter investigation of the role of transjugular intrahepatic portosystemic shunt in the management of portal hypertension. *Radiology* 196:335-340, 1995.

20. Freedman AM, Sanyal AJ, Tisnado J, et al: Complications of trans-jugular intrahepatic portosystemic shunt: A comprehensive review. *Radiographics* 13:1185-1210, 1993.
21. Saxon RR, Ross PL, Mendel-Hartvig J, et al: Transjugular intrahepatic portosystemic shunt patency and the importance of stenosis location in the development of recurrent symptoms. *Radiology* 207:683-693, 1998.
22. LaBerge JM, Ferrell LD, Ring EJ, et al: Histopathologic study of stenotic and occluded transjugular intrahepatic portosystemic shunts. *J Vasc Interv Radiol* 4:779-786, 1993.
23. Pidlich J, Peck-Radosavljevic M, Dranz A, et al: Transjugular intrahepatic portosystemic shunt and cardiac arrhythmias. *J Clin Gastroenterol* 26:39-43, 1998.
24. Warren WD, Restrepo JE, Respess JC, et al: The importance of hemodynamic studies in management of portal hypertension. *Ann Surg* 158:387-404, 1963.
25. Resnick RH, Iber FL, Ishihara AM, et al: A controlled study of the therapeutic portacaval shunt. *Gastroenterology* 67:843-857, 1974.
26. Brophy DP, Haskal ZJ: Simpler ways to deliver the stenotic stent for reducing TIPS flow. *J Vasc Interv Radiol* 9:1032-1033, 1998.
27. Bartorelli AL, Fabbiocchi F, Montorsi P, et al: Successful transcatheter management of Palmaz stent embolization after superior vena cava stenting. *Cathet Cardiovasc Diagn* 34:162-166, 1995.
28. Sanyal AJ, Freedman AM, Purdum PP, et al: The hematologic consequences of transjugular intrahepatic portosystemic shunts. *Hepatology* 23:32-39, 1996.
29. Haskal ZJ, Pentecost MJ, Soulen MC, et al: Transjugular intrahepatic portosystemic shunt stenosis and revision: Early and long term results. *AJR Am J Roentgenol* 163:439-444, 1994.
30. Lind CD, Malisch TW, Chong WK, et al: Incidence of shunt occlusion or stenosis following transjugular intrahepatic portosystemic shunt placement. *Gastroenterology* 106:1277-1283, 1994.
31. Laberge JM, Somberg KA, Lake JR, et al: Two-year outcome following transjugular intrahepatic portosystemic shunt for varical bleeding: Results in 90 patients. *Gastroenterology* 108:1143-1151, 1995
32. Foshager MC, Ferral H, Nazarian GK, et al: Duplex sonography after transjugular intrahepatic portosystemic shunts (TIPS): Normal hemodynamic findings and efficacy in predicting shunt patency and stenosis. *AJR Am J Roentgenol* 165:1-7, 1995.
33. Chong WK, Malisch TW, Mazer MJ: Sonography of transjugular intrahepatic portosystemic shunts. *Semin Ultrasound CT MRI* 16:69-80, 1995.
34. Dodd GD III, Zajko AB, Orons PD, et al: Detection of transjugular intrahepatic portosystemic shunt dysfunction: Value of duplex Doppler sonography. *AJR Am J Roentgenol* 164:1119-1124, 1995.
35. LaBerge JM, Ferrell LD, Ring EJ, et al: Histopathologic study of transjugular intrahepatic portosystemic shunts. *J Vasc Interv Radiol* 2:549-556, 1991.
36. Nishimine K, Saxon RR, Kichikawa K, et al: Improved transjugular

intrahepatic portosystemic shunt patency with PTFE-covered stent-grafts: Experimental results in swine. *Radiology* 196:341-347, 1995.
37. Saxon RR, Timmermans HA, Uchida BT, et al: Stent-grafts for revision of TIPS stenoses and occlusions: A clinical pilot study. *J Vasc Interv Radiol* 8:539-548, 1997.

PART VII
Basic Science

CHAPTER 15

Pharmacologic Inhibition of Aortic Aneurysm Expansion

Michael A. Ricci, M.D.
Associate Professor of Surgery, Division of Vascular and Transplant Surgery, Department of Surgery, University of Vermont College of Medicine, Burlington, Vermont

David B. Pilcher, M.D.
Professor of Surgery, Division of Vascular and Transplant Surgery, Department of Surgery, University of Vermont College of Medicine, Burlington, Vermont

At least 5% of the elderly population of the Western world harbors abdominal aortic aneurysms (AAAs), and the incidence is increasing.[1] Rupture of an AAA is directly related to aneurysm size and results in almost 15,000 deaths per year in the United States.[2] Vascular surgeons generally agree that patients with AAAs larger than 5.0 cm in diameter should be considered for surgical repair, unless there are compelling medical contraindications.[1,3,4] Treatment of smaller aneurysms, those less than 5 cm in size, is more controversial. Although small aneurysms (less than 4.0 cm) rupture infrequently,[5] some surgeons have recommended resection because the AAA will inevitably enlarge with time.[6] Still others[7] have suggested that AAAs less than 5 cm in size are at low risk of rupturing, so they should be followed by serial US measurements. In either situation, however, the pharmacologic inhibition of aneurysm expansion and rupture has never been established.

Although the exact mechanism of AAA formation and expansion is not known, a number of factors have been implicated, including both atherosclerosis[8] and a familial connective tissue abnormality.[9-10] Others have suggested that an imbalance of proteolytic and antiproteolytic activity within the aortic wall is responsible for the expansion and rupture of aortic aneurysms.[11-13] Increased elastase activity, degradation of elastic fibers, and a relative increase in collagen content have all been described in aortic aneurysms.[11-14] More recently, much attention has been focused on the role of the inflammatory response that accompanies aneurysms[15-18] and the tissue or neutrophil enzymes, or matrix metalloproteinases (MMPs), that degrade elastin and collagen.[18] However, the exact sequence in which these changes take place and their ultimate role in the etiology of aneurysm formation is unknown.

BETA-BLOCKADE

Hypertension has also been implicated in the pathogenesis, expansion, and rupture of aortic aneurysms.[19,20] Arterial wall stress is directly proportional to the intraluminal pressure and vessel radius (LaPlace's law). Hypertension increases the arterial tension and, therefore, the risk of rupture.[19,20] Retrospective clinical studies have suggested that hypertension accelerates aneurysm expansion and increases the risk of rupture, as much as 19%.[21,22] Additionally, hypertension increases the rate of rise (dP/dT) of the arterial pressure wave in the aorta, a factor that potentiates the propagating hematoma seen in acute dissecting aneurysms of the aorta.[20,23] The established treatment for this problem is use of the β-adrenergic blockade, which lowers blood pressure (BP) as well as dP/dT, reducing the extent of the dissection and aortic root dilation as well as the risk of aneurysm rupture.[23,24] It is this knowledge that first led to the concept of using β-blockade as a treatment for AAAs.

EXPERIMENTAL EVIDENCE

Evidence from animal models suggests that β-blockade may play a role in stabilizing aneurysms, not only by lowering BP and dP/dT but also by directly affecting aortic elastin.[25-33] Simpson and Boucek[25] investigated drug effects in turkeys fed β-aminopropionitrile fumarate (BAPN), an inhibitor of lysyl oxidase, the enzyme that catalyzes an essential step in the formation of elastin and collagen cross-links, the source of their tensile strength. Broad-breasted white turkeys that spontaneously have hypertension, tachycardia, and atherosclerosis by 5 weeks of age also have dissecting aortic aneurysms when fed BAPN. BAPN has no hemodynamic effects, decreases aortic ring tensile strength, and results in mortality from aneurysm rupture in 44% of turkeys treated with this drug. Animals treated with BAPN and the antihypertensive drug, hydralazine, display lower BP but an increased dP/dT and lower aortic tensile strength, and fatal ruptures occur in 91%. This suggests that factors other than BP reduction affect the aortic wall and the aneurysm rupture rate. BAPN-fed animals treated with nonspecific β-blockade (β$_1$ and β$_2$ receptors) with racemic propranolol had decreased heart rates, BP, and dP/dT, whereas aortic tensile strength increased and the aortic rupture rate fell to 1%. The β$_1$-specific drugs, practolol and sotalol, produced similar hemodynamic effects, but the mortality from ruptures was 13% and 5%, respectively. On the basis of these differences, the authors[25] suggested a direct action on aortic elastin and collagen by propranolol. Other studies from this group have suggested a direct dose–response relationship between propranolol and aortic tensile strength[26] as well as increased cross-linking of elastin with propranolol but not with practolol.[26,27] Although the increase in elastin cross-linking with propranolol was demonstrated by direct measurement of by-products within aortic tissue,[26] the lack of this action by practolol was based only on indirect, histologic evidence.[27]

Studies with a model of elastase-generated aneurysms in rats have suggested that hypertension is associated with the expansion of AAAs.[28] Subsequent studies with this model have suggested that propranolol reduces the expansion of AAAs by a mechanism that may be independent of blood pressure.[20,29] Using the rat model of elastase-induced AAA in normotensive (WKY) and hypertensive (WKHT) rats, investigators studied three groups of animals after induction of AAA formation. Propranolol was administered subcutaneously in two daily doses: 10 mg/kg and 30 mg/kg; control animals received an equivalent volume of saline. The initial tail BP was 129 ± 22 mm Hg in WKY animals and 158 ± 21 mm Hg in WKHT animals ($P < 0.0001$). Tail pressures as well as intra-aortic systolic (sBP), diastolic (dBP), and mean BP were not significantly decreased by propranolol treatment in either strain of rats. The initial aortic size in all animals was 1.06 ± 0.12 mm. At 14 days, the final aortic diameter in untreated, hypertensive rats was more than twice that of untreated normotensive controls: WKY, 3.0 ± 0.73 mm; WKHT, 6.9 ± 3.5 mm; $P < 0.01$. After treatment with both doses of propranolol, aneurysms in hypertensive rats were significantly smaller compared with the untreated WKHT group ($P < 0.05$) and not significantly different from aneurysms in all groups of normotensive animals: WKY$_{10}$, 3.1 ± 1.13 mm; WKHT$_{10}$, 4.0 ± 1.81 mm; WKY$_{30}$, 4.1 ± 0.41 mm; WKHT$_{30}$, 2.9 ± 1.24 mm. There was no significant difference in aortic size between the three normotensive WKY groups. Thus, propranolol treatment was associated with a significant decrease in the size of AAAs in hypertensive animals, which occurs independent of the dose and by a mechanism that may be unrelated to simple BP reduction.[30]

Using the Blotchy mouse, a strain that has abnormally low levels of lysyl oxidase and that has spontaneous aortic aneurysms, Brophy et al.[31] demonstrated that propranolol could delay the formation of aneurysms. Subsequently, these investigators[32] showed increases of 147% in skin elastin and 54% in skin collagen when Blotchy mice were treated with propranolol, which suggests a direct effect on tissue matrix metabolism. However, a recent study,[33] while confirming a reduction in aortic size in Blotchy mice with β-blockade, did not find a parallel increase in lysyl oxidase activity with treatment. Although the heart rate decreased, BP was unaffected, leaving the mechanism of action in doubt.

CLINICAL EVIDENCE

Marfan syndrome, which is characterized by progressive enlargement and eventual rupture of the aortic root, was the subject of a prospective, randomized clinical trial of propranolol.[24] For 10 years, aortic root dimensions and clinical end points (i.e., death, heart failure, aortic dissection, and surgery) were monitored in 32 patients treated with propranolol and in 38 untreated patients. Propranolol was started at 40 mg/day and increased to maintain the heart rate at less than 100 beats/min during exercise. The average subendothelial dose was 212 ± 68 mg/day. Pharmacologic effects were indicated by reductions in heart rate (about 15 beats/min, $P < 0.001$) and BP (at entry: $115/73 \pm 13/10$ mm Hg; at optimal dose: $108/66 \pm 15/11$ mm Hg; sBP: $P = 0.06$; dBP: $P = 0.051$). The regression analysis showed that the slope for the aortic ratio (the ratio of the measured diameter to that predicted from the patient's height, weight, and age) was significantly lower in the treatment group (0.023) compared with controls (0.084; $P < 0.001$). In addition, the survival rate of patients who did not reach a clinical end point was significantly better with propranolol. Two patients in the control group died and four had aortic dissections; no patient in the treatment group died and two noncompliant patients had dissections. The authors concluded that propranolol was successful in reducing the rate of aortic dilation and the associated complications. They also noted that factors other than BP reduction (i.e., negative inotropic and chronotropic effects) may have been responsible for their findings. Unfortunately, decreased aortic dilation and improved survival rates in patients with Marfan syndrome cannot be directly extended to patients with AAAs as the etiology and pathologic process is different.

In a small retrospective study of AAAs, Leach et al.[34] followed 27 patients with AAAs, 12 of whom were receiving β-blocker therapy, over a mean period of 34 months. The expansion rate for the latter group was 0.17 cm/yr compared with those not receiving β-blockers, whose aneurysms grew at a rate of 0.44 cm/yr; however, significance was not attained. Nonetheless, rapid "growth spurts," which they defined as more than 0.32 cm/yr, occurred in only 1 of 12 patients receiving β-blockers (8%) compared with 8 of 15 (53%) not receiving those drugs (*P* = 0.013). They did not report BP control, nor was correlation between BP and the expansion rate done.

A small, retrospective pilot study[35] was carried out at the University of Vermont in 54 patients with AAAs who underwent aortic US over an average of 25.2 months. All antihypertensive medications as well as serial BP measurements were recorded. No correlation between sBP, dBP, or mean BP and expansion rate was found. The mean expansion rate for the entire group was 0.42 ± 0.12 cm/yr. Expansion rates (Table 1) were lowest in patients receiving β-blockers or calcium channel blockers, but the difference was statistically significant only when evaluating calcium channel blockers with the Wilcoxon two-sample nonparametric test.

A subsequent study[36] was reported in which all patients with infrarenal AAAs treated nonoperatively were prospectively followed up during the period 1977-1991 with serial US examinations. Inclusion in the subsequent data analysis required a follow-up period of at least 6 months, at least two US examinations, serial BP determinations, and complete medication histories. AAA size was defined in the sagittal plane only, and it had to be at least 3.0 cm at the time of the first US examination. Patients were divid-

TABLE 1
Abdominal Aortic Aneurysm Expansion Rate

	Expansion Rate			
Drug	**No Medication**	**Taking Medication**	***P* Values**	**Wilcoxon *t* test**
Diuretic (n = 15)	0.38 ± 0.13	0.6 3 ± 0.19	0.27	0.37
Vasodilator (n = 6)	0.42 ± 0.11	0.72 ± 0.38	0.34	0.67
Sympatholytic (n = 5)	0.48 ± 0.12	0.33 ± 0.13	0.66	1.0
β-Blocker (n = 12)	0.57 ± 0.13	0.17 ± 0.14	0.09	0.06
Ca^{2+} Channel Blocker (n = 6)	0.54 ± 0.12	0.04 ± 0.16	0.06	0.01

ed into two groups: patients who did not receive β-blockers during the period of study (group 1) and patients who received β-blockers during the study (group 2). Patients were also classified according to AAA size: 3.0-3.9 cm, 4.0-4.9 cm, and 5.0 cm or larger.

A total of 121 patients were included in the study: 38 were taking β-blockers (group 2). The mean follow-up was 43 ± 29 months with 5.5 ± 3.4 US examinations per patient. The overall expansion rate for the entire population was 0.38 ± 0.44 cm/yr. No correlation was found between expansion rate and age, sex, sBP, dBP, pulse pressure, or mean arterial pressure. Patients in group 1 had an expansion rate of 0.44 ± 0.42 cm/yr compared with group 2 at 0.30 ± 0.31 cm/yr ($P = 0.07$). The number of patients exceeding the mean expansion rate for the entire group (defined as growth spurts by Leach et al.[34]) was significantly greater in group 1 (60%) than in the group receiving β-blockers (19%; $P = 0.03$). Subgroup analysis showed that large aneurysms (5.0 cm or greater) grew significantly faster than smaller aneurysms in group 1 ($P < 0.02$), but this was not seen in group 2 patients. A significant difference in expansion rates between group 1 and group 2 patients with large aneurysms was also seen: 0.68 ± 0.64 cm/yr (group 1) vs. 0.36 ± 0.20 cm/yr (group 2) ($P < 0.05$).

Within group 2, 21 patients were treated with propranolol and the remaining 17 received selective β-blockers (i.e., atenolol or metoprolol). In this small group, the patients treated with propranolol had a significantly slower AAA expansion rate when compared with those patients taking the selective β-blockers: 0.20 ± 0.23 cm/yr vs. 0.42 ± 0.37 cm/yr ($P = 0.03$). A separate analysis of patients taking calcium channel blockers found no significant difference in AAA expansion with those drugs.

A total of 34 patients were followed up with AAAs 5.0 cm or larger because of prohibitive operative risks or the patient's refusal to have surgery. Ten aneurysms that went on to rupture showed a significantly greater expansion rate compared with nonruptured aneurysms in this group: 0.82 ± 0.74 cm/yr vs. 0.42 ± 0.41 cm/yr ($P = 0.04$), which suggests that the rate of expansion may affect the risk of rupture. Eleven patients in group 1 (13%) had AAA ruptures, and two ruptures occurred in group 2 (5%; $P = 0.33$).

This study confirmed that AAAs expand at a greater rate as they enlarge, which is a phenomenon observed by others.[5] Among patients with large AAAs and among those whose AAAs ruptured, the rate of expansion was higher than that of the mean for the entire group, which suggests that rapid expansion may be associated with rupture. Patients taking β-blockers had fewer growth spurts and, in those patients with large AAAs, a significantly slower expansion rate. These effects were most pronounced in patients taking the nonspecific β-blocker propranolol. However, this study was limited by its relatively small size, especially with regard to subgroup analyses. That propranolol did not significantly affect expansion in the overall group, those with small AAAs, or the rupture rate may represent a type II error. Hemodynamic data (beyond BP determinations at the time of clinic visits) were limited, and there was no measure of patient compliance. Acquisition of US images occurred at a number of different hospitals without a standardized protocol (although a single individual reviewed the images). This study was merely observational, and no controlled intervention was carried out. Thus, the effectiveness of propranolol, the groups most likely to benefit, and the overall effect on mortality must be determined by a prospective, randomized, controlled trial before widespread adoption of this therapy can be recommended.

METALLOPROTEINASE INHIBITION

Enzymes capable of degrading elastin include neutrophil elastase and the matrix metalloproteinases MMP-2, MMP-8, MMP-9, and MMP-12 (macrophage metalloelastase). Collagen is the substrate for MMP-1 and MMP-2, which can degrade both collagen and elastin. Those MMPs that have been found in aneurysm tissue, in excess of amounts found in normal or atherosclerotic aortas, include MMP-1, MMP-2, MMP-3, MMP-9, and MMP-12.[18,37-39] In addition, naturally occurring tissue inhibitors of metalloproteinases (TIMPs) may be responsible for maintaining a balance that affects the aortic wall.[40,41]

Much work has been done to investigate the role of MMP-9, which may be the predominant MMP expressed by aortic aneurysm tissue.[40] Tamarina and co-workers[40] found that messenger RNA levels for MMP-9 were 20 times higher than those of MMP-2, whereas TIMP-1 levels were higher than any of the MMPs levels. Others have suggested that elevated MMP-2 levels, particularly in small aneurysms, may play an early role in development of AAAs.[38,41] Still others have suggested a role for an inflammatory mediator, tumor necrosis factor, as a pivotal mediator in the early development of AAAs.[42] These investigators found that tumor necrosis factor–blocking protein was capable of prohibiting the formation of AAAs in the elastase–aneurysm rat model. This work suggests that pharmacologic blockade of the inflammatory response and its mediators is conceivable, particularly early in the course of AAA development.

Because the serine proteases—tissue-type plasminogen activator, urinary-type plasminogen activator, and plasmin—have also been shown to be elevated in AAAs, Allaire and co-workers,[43] in an elegant experiment using a different rat model of AAAs (xenografts in aorta), found that AAA formation and rupture could be prevented when the vessels were seeded with plasminogen activator inhibitor-1 (PAI-1) retrovirally transfected smooth muscle cells. Blocking the plasminogen activator–plasmin pathway with PAI-1 led to the preservation of elastin and decreases in the levels of MMPs. Because AAA rupture in this model was correlated with increased levels of MMP-2 and MMP-9, a second series of experiments investigated the roles of TIMP.[44] Rat smooth muscle cells retrovirally transfected with TIMP-1 DNA were seeded onto the luminal surface of vessels, which resulted in TIMP-1 overexpression. MMP levels were decreased, and aneurysms did not rupture. These authors concluded that pharmacologic inhibition of AAA formation was a reasonable strategy.

INDOMETHACIN

Because aortic aneurysms are accompanied by a histologic inflammatory response within the aortic wall, inhibition of that response might prevent AAA formation. Although blocking of white blood cell attachment in the rat elastase–induced AAA model by anti-CD18 monoclonal antibody demonstrated that AAA formation could be limited, this approach would hardly be practical as a pharmacologic approach in the human. Holmes and colleagues,[45] however, used the anti-inflammatory drug indomethacin in the same elastase-induced rat model of aneurysms. MMP expression is stimulated, in part, by the production of prostaglandin E_2 (PGE_2), which, in turn, is dependent on cyclooxygenase synthetase activity. Because PGE_2 is elevated in AAA tissues, these investigators postulated that AAA could be prevented by blockade of PGE_2 by a cyclooxygenase inhibitor, which, in this experiment, was indomethacin. Although aneurysms developed in five of six control animals, no AAAs developed in those that were treated with 4 mg/kg/day of indomethacin. Although both groups had the characteristic inflammatory response, marked elastin destruction was not present and MMP-9 was decreased in the treated group. Although both of these studies in the same animal model suggest a role for the white blood cells and macrophages, the clinical possibility of using a simple anti-inflammatory agent to block AAA formation, although intriguing, is wholly untested.

DOXYCYCLINE

Tetracyclines inhibit collagenase and MMPs by mechanisms separate from their antibiotic activity.[46,47] They have been demonstrated to be effective in models of gingivitis,[47,48] arthritis,[49] melanomas,[50] and rickets.[51] The mechanism of action, once thought to be the calcium or zinc binding sites on the MMP, seems to be more complex than a simple binding site inhibition alone.[52,53] It may also cause downregulation of cellular MMP production,[53,54] but the mechanism of inhibition of MMPs by tetracycline has not been not clearly elucidated to date.

Petrinec and colleagues[53] investigated the potential of doxycycline to inhibit aneurysm formation in the rat elastase–induced AAA model. Rats treated with doxycycline (25 mg/day subcutaneously) had an 8% incidence of aneurysm formation (defined as a twofold increase in aortic size) compared with 83% in controls ($P < 0.01$). Doxycycline prevented the degradation of elastin within the aortic wall and decreased the production of MMP-9, yet it did not attenuate the inflammatory response. Thus, decreased production of MMP-9, normally produced in aneurysms by macrophages, occurred in spite of the inflammatory response. This led to the conclusion that production of MMP-9 is inhibited directly or at the level of cellular production, and local production of MMP-9 is a necessary step in the formation of aneurysms in this model. However, because doxycycline inhibits a number of MMPs and they were not measured in this study, the possibility remains that another pathway or MMP may be directly responsible for the lack of aneurysm expansion in this model. These research groups have found similar results with four different, nonantibiotic, chemically modified tetracycline derivatives as well.[55]

Boyle and co-workers[56] used an in vitro model of aneurysm formation. Porcine aortic segments were cultured with elastase, which produces the typical histologic appearance of aortic degradation in the aortic tissue. When cultured with doxycycline, elastin was preserved. MMP-9 production was decreased, which confirmed the in vivo work done by Petrinec and colleagues.[53] In addition, these authors found that production of MMP-2, as well as TIMP-1 and TIMP-2, was not altered by doxycycline. Again, however, inhibition of MMPs is suggested by these two studies as a means of potentially retarding aneurysm formation or expansion. The authors point out that tetracyclines have a large margin of safety, and long-term administration has been tested by time in other disease states, notably acne.[56]

CONCLUSION

Experimental evidence seems to strongly suggest that pharmacologic suppression of the growth of aneurysms is possible yet still unproved. The most evidence has been accumulated to date about β-blockers. So far, this suggests that β-blockers, in general, and propranolol, in particular, exert effects that delay the onset, limit expansion, and reduce the risk of rupture of aneurysms in three different animal models. Propranolol is superior to other antihypertensive agents as well as selective β-blockers in producing these effects. It may exert a direct effect on elastin cross-linking within the aorta, resulting in greater tensile strength. However, it is likely that the mechanism of action is multifactorial, including both tissue protein effects as well as hemodynamic effects. Clinical studies have shown promise, but conclusions regarding their findings must be interpreted with caution because of small numbers or design problems.

One of the key questions not yet answered is whether a slower expansion rate will reduce the need for surgery and the risk of rupture or merely delay surgery or rupture. An ongoing clinical trial in Canada may provide an answer.

Other methods that have potential may include anti-inflammatory agents or tetracyclines or both. Obviously, the latter, with their high safety profile, are most attractive. However, to date, there are no clinical data on which to base any judgment.

Pharmacologic inhibition of aortic aneurysms engenders many questions. One of the clear problems with pharmacologic inhibition relates to timing of the administration of any of these agents. When does one start the drug? Should high-risk patients (e.g., those with family histories, those who smoke, those who are elderly) have treatment? Is it too late once an aneurysm is detected? Is there a role only for small aneurysms, or do large, inoperable AAAs have one as well? Will treatment with these agents ultimately produce a worse quality of life or lead to other complications? Given these questions and that current practice seems to be swinging toward earlier repair of AAAs or the use of new endovascular technologies to treat small AAAs, there is an immediate need for a randomized, controlled clinical trial to determine the best medical management of aortic aneurysms.

REFERENCES

1. Hollier LH, Taylor LM, Oschner J: Recommended indications for operative treatment of abdominal aortic aneurysms. *J Vasc Surg* 15:1046-1056, 1992.
2. National Center for Health Statistics: *Vital Statistics of the United States, 1988, Mortality, Part A*, vol 2. Washington, DC: Government Printing Office, DHHS publication No PHS 91-1101, 1991.
3. Pilcher DB, Davis JH: Aorta and peripheral arteries, in Davis JH (ed): *Clinical Surgery*. St Louis, CV Mosby, 1987, pp 2094-2167.
4. Ernst CB: Current concepts: Abdominal aortic aneurysms. *N Eng J Med* 328:1167-1172, 1993.
5. Nevitt MP, Ballard DJ, Hallett JW Jr: Prognosis of abdominal aortic aneurysms: A population based study. *N Eng J Med* 321:1009-1014, 1989.

6. Cronenwett JL, Sargent SK, Wall MH, et al: Variables that affect the expansion rate and outcome of small abdominal aortic aneurysms. *J Vasc Surg* 11:260-269, 1990.

7. Bernstein EF, Chan EL: Abdominal aortic aneurysm in high-risk patients: Outcome of selective management based on size and expansion rate. *Ann Surg* 200:255-263, 1984.

8. Zarins CK, Glagov S, Vesselinovitch D, et al: Aneurysm formation in experimental atherosclerosis: Relationship to plaque evolution. *J Vasc Surg* 12:246-256, 1990.

9. Tilson MD, Seashore MR: Fifty families with abdominal aortic aneurysms in two or more first-order relatives. *Am J Surg* 147:551-553, 1984.

10. Johansen K, Koepsell T: Familial tendency for abdominal aortic aneurysms. *JAMA* 256:1934-1936, 1986.

11. Menashi S, Campa JS, Greenhalgh RM, et al: Collagen in abdominal aortic aneurysm: Typing, content, and degradation. *J Vasc Surg* 6:578-582, 1987.

12. Cohen JR, Mandell C, Margolis I, et al: Altered aortic protease and antiprotease activity in patients with ruptured abdominal aortic aneurysms. *Surg Gynecol Obstet* 164:355-358, 1987.

13. Cohen JR, Mandell C, Chang JB, et al: Elastin metabolism of the infrarenal aorta. *J Vasc Surg* 7:210-214, 1988.

14. Baxter BT, McGee GS, Shively VP, et al: Elastin content, cross-links, and mRNA in normal and aneurysmal human aorta. *J Vasc Surg* 16:192-200, 1992.

15. Koch AE, Haines GK, Rizzo RJ, et al: Human abdominal aortic aneurysms. Immunophenotypic analysis suggesting an immune-related response. *Am J Pathol* 137:1199-1213, 1990.

16. Anidjar S, Dobrin PB, Eichorst M, et al: Correlation of inflammatory infiltrate with the enlargement of experimental aortic aneurysms. *J Vasc Surg* 16:139-147, 1992.

17. Ricci MA, Strindberg G, Slaiby JM, et al: Anti-CD18 monoclonal antibody slows experimental aortic aneurysm expansion. *J Vasc Surg* 23:301-307, 1996.

18. Rehm JP, Grange JJ, Baxter BT: The formation of aneurysms. *Semin Vasc Surg* 11:192-202, 1998.

19. Spittell JA Jr: Hypertension and arterial aneurysm. *J Am Coll Cardiol* 1:533-540, 1983.

20. Dobrin PB: Pathophysiology and pathogenesis of aortic aneurysms. *Surg Clin North Am* 69:687-703, 1989.

21. Szilagyi DE, Elliott JP, Smith RF: Clinical fate of the patient with asymptomatic abdominal aortic aneurysm unfit for surgical treatment. *Arch Surg* 104:600-606, 1972.

22. Cronenwett JL, Murphy TF, Zelenock GB, et al: Actuarial analysis of variables associated with rupture of small abdominal aortic aneurysms. *Surgery* 98:472-483, 1985.

23. Wheat MW Jr: Acute dissecting aneurysms of the aorta: Diagnosis and treatment—1979. *Am Heart J* 99:373-387, 1980.

24. Shores J, Berger KR, Murphy EA, et al: Progression of aortic dilation and the benefit of long-term β-adrenergic blockade in Marfan's Syndrome. *N Eng J Med* 330:1335-1341, 1994.

25. Simpson CF, Boucek RJ: The β-aminopropionitrile-fed turkey: A model for detecting potential drug action on arterial tissue. *Cardiovasc Res* 17:26-32, 1983.

26. Boucek RJ, Gunja-Smith Z, Noble NL, et al: Modulation by propranolol of the lysyl cross-links in aortic elastin and collagen of the aneurysm-prone turkey. *Biochem Pharmacol* 32:275-280, 1983.

27. Simpson CF, Boucek RJ, Noble NL: Influence of *d-*, *l-*, and *dl*-propranolol, and practolol on β-aminopropionitrile-induced aortic rupture of turkeys. *Toxicol Appl Pharmacol* 38:169-175, 1976.

28. Gadowski GR, Ricci MA, Hendley ED, et al: Hypertension accelerates the growth of experimentally induced abdominal aortic aneurysms. *J Surg Res* 54:431-436, 1993.

29. Slaiby J, Ricci MA, Gadowski G, et al: Propranolol reduces the size of aortic aneurysms in hypertensive rats. *Surg Forum* 44:343-344, 1993.

30. Slaiby JM, Ricci MA, Gadowski GR, et al: Growth of aortic aneurysms is reduced by propranolol in a hypertensive rat model. *J Vasc Surg* 20:178-183, 1994.

31. Brophy CM, Tilson JE, Tilson MD: Propranolol delays the formation of aneurysms in the male Blotchy mouse. *J Surg Res* 44:687-691, 1988.

32. Brophy CM, Tilson JE, Tilson MD: Propranolol stimulates the cross-linking of matrix components in skin from the aneurysm-prone Blotchy mouse. *J Surg Res* 46:330-332, 1989.

33. Moursi MM, Beebe HG, Messina LM, et al: Inhibition of aortic aneurysm development in Blotchy mice by beta-adrenergic blockade independent of altered lysyl oxidase activity. *J Vasc Surg* 21:792-800, 1995.

34. Leach SD, Toole AL, Stern H, et al: Effect of β-adrenergic blockade on the growth rate of abdominal aortic aneurysms. *Arch Surg* 123:606-609, 1988.

35. Pilcher DB, unpublished data, 1988.

36. Gadowski GR, Pilcher DB, Ricci MA: Abdominal aortic aneurysm expansion rate: Effect of size and beta-adrenergic blockade. *J Vasc Surg* 19:727-731, 1994.

37. Thompson RW, Holmes DR, Mertens RA, et al: Production and localization of 92-kilodalton gelatinase in abdominal aortic aneurysms: An elastolytic metalloproteinase expressed by aneurysm-infiltrating macrophages. *J Clin Invest* 96:318-326, 1995.

38. Freestone T, Turner RJ, Coady A, et al: Inflammation and matrix metalloproteinases in the enlarging abdominal aortic aneurysm. *Arterioscler Thromb Vasc Biol* 15:1145-1151, 1995.

39. Davis V, Persidskaia R, Baca-Regen L, et al: Matrix metalloproteinase-2 production and its binding to the matrix are increased in abdominal aortic aneurysms. *Arterioscler Thromb Vasc Biol* 18:1625-1633, 1998.

40. Tamarina NA, McMillan WD, Shively VP, et al: Expression of matrix metalloproteinases and their inhibitors in aneurysms and normal aorta. *Surgery* 122:264-271, 1997.

41. Grange JJ, Davis V, Baxter BT: Pathogenesis of abdominal aortic aneurysm: An update and look toward the future. *Cardiovasc Surg* 5:256-265, 1997.
42. Hingorani A, Ascher E, Scheinman M, et al: The effect of tumor necrosis factor binding protein and interleukin-1 receptor antagonist on the development of abdominal aortic aneurysms in a rat model. *J Vasc Surg* 28:522-526, 1998.
43. Allaire E, Forough R, Clowes M, et al: Local overexpression of TIMP-1 prevents aortic aneurysm degeneration and rupture in a rat model. *J Clin Invest* 102:1413-1420, 1998.
44. Allaire E, Hasenstab D, Kenagy RD, et al: Prevention of aneurysm development and rupture by local overexpression of plasminogen activator inhibitor-1. *Circulation* 98:249-255, 1998.
45. Holmes DR, Petrinec D, Webster W, et al: Indomethacin prevents elastase-induced abdominal aortic aneurysms in the rat. *J Surg Res* 63:305-309, 1996.
46. Golub LM, Ramamurthy S, McNamara TF, et al: Tetracyclines inhibit connective tissue breakdown: New therapeutic implications for an old family of drugs. *Crit Rev Oral Biol Med* 2:297-321, 1991.
47. Ryan ME, Ramamurthy S, Golub LM: Matrix metalloproteinases and their inhibition in periodontal treatment. *Curr Opin Periodontol* 3:85-96, 1996.
48. Golub LM, Lee HM, Greenwald RA, et al: A matrix metalloproteinase inhibitor reduces bone-type collagen degradation fragments and specific collagenases in gingival crevicular fluid during adult periodontitis. *Inflamm Res* 46:310-319, 1997.
49. Zernicke RF, Wohl GR, Greenwald RA, et al: Administration of systemic matrix metalloproteinase inhibitors maintains bone mechanical integrity in adjuvant arthritis. *J Rheumatol* 24:1324-1331, 1997.
50. Seftor RE, Seftor EA, De Larco JE, et al: Chemically modified tetracyclines inhibit human melanoma cell invasion and metastasis. *Clin Exp Metastasis* 16:217-225, 1998.
51. Greenwald RA, Simonson BG, Moak SA, et al: Inhibition of epiphyseal cartilage collagenase by tetracyclines in low phosphate rickets in rats. *J Orthop Res* 6:695-703, 1988.
52. Sorsa T, Ramamurthy S, Vernillo AT, et al: Functional sites of chemically modified tetracyclines: Inhibition of the oxidative activation of human neutrophil and chicken osteoclast pro-matrix metalloproteinases. *J Rheumatol* 25:975-982, 1998.
53. Petrinec D, Shixiong L, Holmes DR, et al: Doxycycline inhibition of aneurysmal degeneration in an elastase-induced rat model of abdominal aortic aneurysm: Preservation of aortic elastin associated with suppressed production of 92 kD gelantinase. *J Vasc Surg* 23:336-346, 1996.
54. Uitto VJ, Firth JD, Nip L, et al: Doxycycline and chemically-modified tetracyclines inhibit gelatinase (MMP-2) gene expression in human skin keratinocytes. *Ann N Y Acad Sci* 732:140-151, 1994.
55. Curci JA, Petrinec D, Liao S, et al: Pharmacologic suppression of experimental abdominal aortic aneurysms: A comparison of doxycy-

cline and four chemically modified tetracyclines. *J Vasc Surg* 28:1082-1093, 1998.

56. Boyle JR, McDermott E, Crowther M, et al: Doxycycline inhibits elastin degradation and reduces metalloproteinase activity in a model of aneurysm disease. *J Vasc Surg* 27:354-361, 1998.

Index

A

Abciximab, 186
Abdominal pain, after transjugular
    intrahepatic portosystemic
    shunt, 213
ACAS criteria, for duplex
    scanning of internal carotid
    artery stenosis, 49-50
Age of asymptomatic patients
    undergoing carotid
    endarterectomy
co-morbidity and, 33-34
death and
    late, 30
    perioperative, 29
outcome and, 31-32
stroke and, perioperative, 28
Air emboli, and carbon dioxide
    insufflation for vascular
    surgery, 133
Alopecia, after long-term heparin
    usage, 182
Ancrod, 185-186
 in heparin-induced
    thrombocytopenia and
    thrombosis syndrome, 182
AnCure graft for endovascular
    repair of abdominal aortic
    aneurysms
attachment system, 89, 90, 91
features, 90
Anesthesia
 in carotid endarterectomy,
    eversion, 72, 73
general, in transjugular
    intrahepatic portosystemic
    shunting, 206, 213
AneuR$_x$ graft, for endovascular
    repair of abdominal aortic
    aneurysms, features of, 90
Aneurysm
aortic, abdominal

expansion, beta-blockade
    inhibition of (see Beta-
    blockade inhibition of aortic
    aneurysm expansion)
expansion, doxycycline
    inhibition of, 236-237
expansion, indomethacin
    inhibition of, 236
expansion, metalloproteinase
    inhibition of, 235-237
expansion, pharmacologic
    inhibition of, 229-242
expansion, rate, 233
repair, endovascular graft for
    (see Endovascular, graft for
    abdominal aortic aneurysm
    repair)
repair, laparoscopic (see
    Laparoscopy, abdominal
    aortic aneurysm repair by)
splenic artery, laparoscopic
    ligation of, 124
Angina, unstable, low-molecular
    weight heparin in, 184-185
Angiography
completion digital subtraction, of
    endoleak, 112
contrast, in diagnosis of carotid
    kinks and coils, 79
CT
    of endoleak after endovascular
        repair of abdominal aortic
        aneurysm, 113
    of endoleak after endovascular
        repair of abdominal aortic
        aneurysm, in follow-up, 120
    helical, of endoleak after
        endovascular repair of
        abdominal aortic aneurysm,
        119
    after Wallstent placement for
        endoleaks, 111

Angioplasty
patch, in carotid endarterectomy
eversion, 57
vs. primary closure (*see*
Endarterectomy, carotid,
closure, primary *vs.* patch
angioplasty)
percutaneous transluminal, *vs.*
exercise therapy for
claudication, 148, 162-163
ankle-brachial indices after, 162
walking distance after, 163
Angioscope in endovascular in
situ bypass, 138
in retracted position, 140
Angioscopic imaging, of side branch
orifice in endovascular in situ
bypass, 140
Ankle-brachial indices, after
exercise therapy *vs.*
percutaneous transluminal
angioplasty for claudication,
162
Anorectal variceal bleeding, shunt
for (*see* Shunt, portosystemic,
transjugular intrahepatic)
Anticoagulants
compounds related to, listing of,
180
listing of, 180
old and new, 179-188
Anticoagulation for infrainguinal
revascularization, 167-178
effect on long-term graft patency,
170-174
in immediate postoperative
period, 170
to improve early graft patency,
168-170
long-term usage, current
approach to, 174-176
Antiplatelet agents, 186
effect on early graft patency after
infrainguinal
revascularization, 168-169

in heparin-induced
thrombocytopenia and
thrombosis syndrome, 182
Aortic
aneurysm (*see* Aneurysm, aortic)
bypass, laparoscopic (in pig), 125
para-aortic lymph node biopsy,
laparoscopic, 124
replacement, sutureless
prosthesis for, 134
Aortobifemoral bypass,
laparoscopic-assisted, 124
Argatroban, 185
in heparin-induced
thrombocytopenia and
thrombosis syndrome, 182
Arrhythmia, after portosystemic
shunt placement, transjugular
intrahepatic, 218
Arteriogram, completion, after
endovascular
femoroposterior tibial in situ
bypass, 142
Artery
carotid (*see* Carotid)
claudication (*see* Claudication)
iliac, right internal, cannulation
and coil embolization prior
to endograft repair of
abdominal aortic aneurysm,
95
iliolumbar, coil embolization, for
treatment of endoleak after
endovascular repair of
abdominal aortic aneurysm,
116
puncture during transjugular
intrahepatic portosystemic
shunt placement, 216
splenic, aneurysm, laparoscopic
ligation of, 124
Arvin, 185-186
in heparin-induced
thrombocytopenia and
thrombosis syndrome, 182

Ascites, massive intractable, shunt
for (*see* Shunt,
portosystemic, transjugular
intrahepatic)
Aspirin, 186
/dipyridamole, effect on early
graft patency after
infrainguinal
revascularization, 168-169
in heparin-induced
thrombocytopenia and
thrombosis syndrome, 182
in infrainguinal revascularization
effect on long-term graft
patency, 171
long-term usage, 174-175
/warfarin in infrainguinal
revascularization, 174-176
effect on long-term graft
patency, 172
Atenolol, inhibition of aortic
aneurysm expansion by, 234
Atrial arrhythmia, after
portosystemic shunt
placement, transjugular
intrahepatic, 218

B

Baxter graft, for endovascular
repair of abdominal aortic
aneurysms, features of, 90
Beta-blockade inhibition of aortic
aneurysm expansion, 230-235
clinical evidence, 232-235
experimental evidence, 230-232
Bifurcationplasty, carotid
advancement, 70
Biliary
complications after portosystemic
shunt placement, transjugular
intrahepatic, 216-217, 217-218
-venous fistula, occluded stent
related to, after transjugular
intrahepatic portosystemic
shunt placement, 217

Biopsy, lymph node, laparoscopic
para-aortic, 124
Bleeding
control in laparoscopic surgery
for abdominal aortic
aneurysms, 133
gastrointestinal, recurrent upper,
after transjugular
intrahepatic portosystemic
shunt, 215
heparin causing, standard
unfractionated, 181-182
hirudin causing, 185
variceal, shunt for (*see* Shunt,
portosystemic, transjugular
intrahepatic)
Brown vascular exercise program
for claudication (*see*
Exercise, program for
claudication, supervised,
Brown)
Budd-Chiari syndrome, stenting to
inferior vena cava in, 204
Bypass
aortic, laparoscopic (in pig),
125
aortobifemoral, laparoscopic-
assisted, 124
endovascular in situ, 137-146
angioscope in, 138
angioscope in retracted
position in, 140
arteriogram after, completion,
142
coil delivery catheter in, 141
cost data, 145
Gianturco coil deployed from
coil delivery catheter in, 141
hospital length of stay after,
145
patency rates at 36 months'
follow-up, 144
performed through two
incisions, 143
side branch in, embolized, 141

side branch occlusion in,
  technique, 139-146
side branch orifice in,
  angioscopic imaging of, 140
technique of operation, 138-146
valvulotome cutting blade
  extended in, 139
valvulotomy in, technique,
  138-139
graft, lower extremity, reasons
  why patients have grafts at
  high risk for failure and/or
  limb loss, 175
infrainguinal, anticoagulation for
  (*see* Anticoagulation for
  infrainguinal
  revascularization)

C

Carbon dioxide
  insufflation for vascular surgery,
    and air emboli, 133
  portography, hepatic wedge, for
    portal vein localization for
    transjugular intrahepatic
    portosystemic shunt,
    206-208
Cardiac (*see* Heart)
Care
  intensive care unit, duration of
    stay after laparoscopic
    abdominal aortic aneurysm
    repair, 132
  postprocedural, after transjugular
    intrahepatic portosystemic
    shunt, 212-215
Carotid
  artery
    common, redundant, plication
      of, 83
    internal (*see below*)
    kinks and coils (*see* Kinks and
      coils of carotid artery)
    nonredundant, in eversion
      endarterectomy, 70

occlusive disease, spectral
  analysis of, 41-53
restenosis after carotid
  endarterectomy with greater
  saphenous vein patching *vs.*
  synthetic patching and
  everted cervical vein
  patching, 17
stenosis (*see* Stenosis, carotid
  artery)
artery, internal
  occlusion, early postoperative,
    after primary *vs.* patch
    angioplasty closure after
    carotid endarterectomy, 11
  plaque, elevation in eversion
    endarterectomy, 63
  reanastomosis to common
    carotid in eversion
    endarterectomy, 67
  redundant, excision, in
    eversion endarterectomy, 62
  shortening, combined with
    endarterectomy for kinks
    and coils, 81-82
  shortening, combined with
    endarterectomy for kinks and
    coils, plication of redundant
    common carotid in, 83
  transection in eversion
    endarterectomy, 61
  bifurcationplasty, advancement, 70
  endarterectomy (*see*
    Endarterectomy, carotid)
Catheter, coil delivery, in
  endovascular in situ bypass,
  141
Cervical vein patches, everted, *vs.*
  saphenous vein closure after
  carotid endarterectomy,
  15-18
Children, carotid kinks and coils
  in
  etiology, 78
  incidence, 78

Cilostazol, for claudication, 161
Claudication
    drug therapy for, 160-161
    exercise program for (*see*
        Exercise program for
        claudication)
    exercise therapy for (*see* Exercise
        therapy for claudication)
    natural history, 160
Clopidogrel, 186
    effect on long-term graft patency
        after infrainguinal
        revascularization, 171-172
CO_2 portography, hepatic wedge,
        for portal vein localization
        for transjugular intrahepatic
        portosystemic shunt, 206-208
Coagulation, basis of, 179-181
Coil(s)
    carotid (*see* Kinks and coils of
        carotid artery)
    delivery catheter in endovascular
        in situ bypass, 141
    embolization
        iliac artery, right internal, prior
            to endograft repair of
            abdominal aortic aneurysm,
            95
        iliolumbar artery, for treatment
            of endoleak after
            endovascular repair of
            abdominal aortic aneurysm,
            116
        Gianturco, deployed from coil
            delivery catheter in
            endovascular in situ bypass,
            141
Co-morbidity and carotid
        endarterectomy for
        asymptomatic patients, 24-25
    age and, 33-34
    endarterectomy outcome and, 31
    impact on death
        late, 30
        perioperative, 29

impact on perioperative stroke, 28
Computed tomography (*see* CT)
Contrast
    angiography in diagnosis of
        carotid kinks and coils, 79
    material, iodinated, in
        transjugular intrahepatic
        portosystemic shunt
        placement, complications of,
        221
Corvita graft, for endovascular
        repair of abdominal aortic
        aneurysms, features of, 90
Cost
    of endovascular in situ bypass,
        145
    of heparin, low-molecular
        weight, for treatment of
        venous thromboembolism,
        184
CT
    angiography (*see* Angiography,
        CT)
    of endoleak, distal attachment
        site, after endovascular
        repair of abdominal aortic
        aneurysm, 101
    follow-up
        of endoleak, distal attachment
            site, after endovascular graft
            repair of abdominal aortic
            aneurysm, 101
        after endovascular repair of
            abdominal aortic aneurysm,
            100

D

Dacron
    as endovascular graft material for
        repair of abdominal aortic
        aneurysms, 92
    patch *vs.* autologous greater
        saphenous vein closure in
        carotid endarterectomy,
        15-18

Danaparoid sodium, in heparin-
    induced thrombocytopenia
    and thrombosis syndrome,
    182
Death (*see* Mortality)
Decision making, for asymptomatic
    patients with critical carotid
    stenosis, 23-39
Demographics, in eversion carotid
    endarterectomy, 72
Dextran, effect on early graft
    patency after infrainguinal
    revascularization, 169
Dicumarol, in infrainguinal
    revascularization, effect on
    long-term graft patency, 172
Diet, clear liquid, interval to
    tolerating, after laparoscopic
    abdominal aortic aneurysm
    repair, 131
Dipyridamole, 186
  /aspirin, effect on early graft
    patency after infrainguinal
    revascularization, 168-169
Doppler ultrasound (*see*
    Ultrasound, Doppler)
Doxycycline, inhibition of aortic
    aneurysm expansion by,
    236-237
Drug(s)
  antiplatelet
    effect on early graft patency
      after infrainguinal
      revascularization, 168-169
    in heparin-induced
      thrombocytopenia and
      thrombosis syndrome, 182
  therapy for claudication, 160-161
Duplex scanning (*see* Ultrasound,
    duplex)

E

Education lectures, in Brown
    vascular exercise program
    for claudication, 154

Embolism
  air, and carbon dioxide
    insufflation for vascular
    surgery, 133
  pulmonary, low-molecular
    weight heparin in, 184
Embolization
  coil
    of iliac artery, right internal,
      prior to endograft repair of
      abdominal aortic aneurysm,
      95
    of iliolumbar artery, for
      treatment of endoleak after
      endovascular repair of
      abdominal aortic aneurysm,
      116
  of side branch in endovascular
    in situ bypass, 141
Encephalopathy
  poorly controlled, as
    contraindication to
    transjugular intrahepatic
    portosystemic shunts, 201
  after portosystemic shunt
    placement, transjugular
    intrahepatic, 214, 218-219
Endarterectomy, carotid
  in asymptomatic patients, 23-39
  characteristics of patient
    sample, 26
  clinical relevance of age and
    co-morbidity, 33-34
  death after, late, impact of age,
    sex, race, and co-morbidity
    on, 30
  death after, perioperative,
    impact of age, sex, race, and
    co-morbidity on, 29
  follow-up, long-term, 28-30
  future prospects, 36-37
  impact of co-morbidity, 24-25
  impact of demographics, 24-25
  impact of prospective
    randomized trials, 23-24

morbidity of, perioperative, 26-28

mortality of, perioperative, 26-28

outcome, and age, 31-32

outcome, and cardiac disease, 30-31

outcome, and other co-morbidities, 31

outcome, effect of hospital and surgeon case volume on, 34-36

stroke after, perioperative, impact of age, sex, race, and co-morbidity on, 28

closure, primary *vs.* patch angioplasty, 8-10

early internal carotid occlusion after, 11

effect of patch material on outcomes, 14-18

outcomes, 10-13

practical and theoretical advantages of patch reconstruction, 13-14

restenosis after, 13

stroke after, 12

combined with shortening of internal carotid for kinks and coils, 81-82

plication of redundant common carotid in, 83

death rates in, 3-6

eversion, 55-76

clinical materials, 71-74

demographics, 72

elevation of internal carotid plaque in, 63

excision of redundant internal carotid artery in, 62

of external and common carotid arteries, 66

indications for, 72

methods, 58-71

nonredundant carotids in, 70

operative parameters, 73

patency and patient survival rates, cumulative, 74

perioperative management, 59-60

plaque removal and visualization of end point in, 64

reanastomosis of internal to common carotid artery in, 67

reanastomosis with shunt in place in, 69

results, 71-74

selection of cases, 58-59

shunt use in, 68-69

technical suggestions, 70-71

technique, 60-67

transection of internal carotid artery in, 61

outcomes, 1-22

individual surgeon, 6-8

stroke in, perioperative, 3-6

technique of, changing, 71

Endoleaks after endovascular repair of abdominal aortic aneurysms, 98, 105-122

angiogram of, completion digital subtraction, 112

case descriptions, 109-116

classification, 99

by source, 106

coil embolization for, iliolumbar artery, 116

consequences of, 107

distal attachment site, on follow-up CT, 101

treatment

authors' approach to, 119-120

follow-up imaging, 118-119

how and when, 105-122

what is known about, 116-118

unpredictability of, 107-109

Endovascular

graft for abdominal aortic aneurysm repair, 87-104

attachment systems, 89-92
characteristics, 89-94
complications, 96-103
delivery systems, 93-94
deployment systems, 94
endoleaks after (*see*
    Endoleaks)
follow-up, CT, 100
historical perspective, 88-89
limb dysfunction after,
    Wallstent for, 102, 103
material for, 92
modular *vs.* single-unit design,
    92-93
results, 96, 97
selection of patients for, 94-95
support systems, 92
technical success and mortality,
    96
in situ bypass (*see* Bypass,
    endovascular in situ)
Equipment requirements, for
    Brown vascular exercise
    program for claudication,
    149
Excluder graft for endovascular
    repair of abdominal aortic
    aneurysms
features, 90
illustration, 93
Exercise program for claudication,
    supervised, 147-166
Brown
    cardiac screening before, 151
    components, 149-150
    education lectures in, 154
    equipment requirements, 149
    exercise sessions in, 153-154
    nursing evaluation before,
        150-151
    patient population, 155
    personnel requirements,149
    phase 1, 150-153
    phase 2, 153-154
    phase 3, 155

quality of life measurements
    after, 157-159
resources for, 149-150
results, 155-160
space for, 149-150
structure, 150-155
treadmill testing before,
    progressive, 151-153
vascular testing before,
    noninvasive, 151
walking ability after,
    155-157
reimbursement for, 159-160
starting a program, 159
Exercise therapy for claudication,
    161-163
supervised program of (*see*
    Exercise program for
    claudication, supervised
    above)
vs. angioplasty, percutaneous
    transluminal
ankle-brachial indices after,
    162
walking distance after, 163
Extremity
dysfunction after endovascular
    graft repair of abdominal
    aortic aneurysm, Wallstent
    for, 100, 101
lower, bypass grafts, at high risk
    for failure and/or limb loss,
    reasons why patients have,
    175
Extubation, after laparoscopic
    abdominal aortic aneurysm
    repair, hours to, 131

F

Femoroposterior tibial in situ
    bypass, endovascular
completion arteriogram after,
    142
performed through two
    incisions, 143

Fistula, biliary-venous, relation to stent occlusion after transjugular intrahepatic portosystemic shunt placement, 217

Flow phantom for three-dimensional ultrasound, 196
coronal view of, 197

Fogarty valvulotome in endovascular in situ bypass, 137, 138
cutting blade extended, illustration, 139

G

Gastroesophageal variceal bleeding, shunt for (*see* Shunt, portosystemic, transjugular intrahepatic)

Gastrointestinal bleeding, recurrent upper, after transjugular intrahepatic portosystemic shunt, 215

Gianturco coil, deployed from coil delivery catheter in endovascular in situ bypass, 141

Graft
bypass, lower extremity, reasons why patients have grafts at high risk for failure and/or limb loss, 175
endovascular, for abdominal aortic aneurysm repair (*see* Endovascular, graft for abdominal aortic aneurysm repair)

H

Heart
compromise, right-sided, as contraindication to transjugular intrahepatic portosystemic shunts, 201
disease, and carotid endarterectomy outcome in asymptomatic patients, 30-31
failure, congestive, and outcome of carotid endarterectomy in asymptomatic patients, 30-31
screening before Brown vascular exercise program for claudication, 151

Hemobilia, after portosystemic shunt placement, transjugular intrahepatic, 216

Hemolytic syndrome, transient, after portosystemic shunt placement, transjugular intrahepatic, 219

Heparin
in carotid endarterectomy, eversion, 61
in infrainguinal revascularization effect on early graft patency, 169
in immediate postoperative period, 170
low-molecular weight, 183-185
in heparin-induced thrombocytopenia and thrombosis syndrome, 182
in infrainguinal revascularization, effect on early graft patency, 170
in infrainguinal revascularization, in immediate postoperative period, 170
prophylactic, after portosystemic shunt placement, transjugular intrahepatic, 214
standard unfractionated, 181-183
mechanism of action, 181

Hepatic
(*See also* Liver)
hydrothorax, shunt for (*see*
    Shunt, portosystemic,
    transjugular intrahepatic)
intrahepatic portosystemic
    shunt, transjugular (see
    Shunt, portosystemic,
    transjugular intrahepatic)
vein stenosis, delayed, after
    transjugular intrahepatic
    portosystemic shunt
    placement, 220
wedge portography with CO_2 for
    portal vein localization for
    transjugular intrahepatic
    portosystemic shunt,
    206-208
Hip surgery, orthopedic, low-
    molecular weight heparin in,
    184
Hirudin, 185
Hirulog, 185
Hospital
case volume, effect on outcome
    of carotid endarterectomy in
    asymptomatic patients,
    34-36
length of stay
    after endovascular in situ
        bypass, 145
    after laparoscopic abdominal
        aortic aneurysm repair,
        132
Hydrothorax, hepatic, shunt for
    (*see* Shunt, portosystemic,
    transjugular intrahepatic)
Hypertension, pulmonary, as
    contraindication to
    transjugular intrahepatic
    shunts, 201
Hypotension, mild arterial, after
    portosystemic shunt
    placement, transjugular
    intrahepatic, 213

I

ICU, duration of stay after
    laparoscopic abdominal
    aortic aneurysm repair, 132
Iliac artery, right internal,
    cannulation and coil
    embolization prior to
    endograft repair of
    abdominal aortic aneurysm,
    95
Iliolumbar artery, coil
    embolization, for treatment
    of endoleak after
    endovascular repair of
    abdominal aortic aneurysm,
    116
Imaging
angioscopic, of side branch
    orifice in endovascular in
    situ bypass, 140
color Doppler energy, 191
follow-up, of endoleaks after
    endovascular repair of
    abdominal aortic aneurysms,
    118-119
Incisions, two, for endovascular in
    situ bypass, 143
Indomethacin, 186
inhibition of aortic aneurysm
    expansion by, 236
Infectious complications, of
    portosystemic shunt
    placement, transjugular
    intrahepatic, 220
Infrainguinal revascularization
ancrod in, 185
anticoagulation for (*see*
    Anticoagulation for
    infrainguinal
    revascularization)
Instrument passage, transcapsular,
    during transjugular
    intrahepatic portosystemic
    shunt placement, 216

Intensive care unit, duration of
stay after laparoscopic
abdominal aortic aneurysm
repair, 132
Intrahepatic portosystemic shunt,
transjugular (*see* Shunt,
portosystemic, transjugular
intrahepatic)
Intravascular ultrasound, in
carotid stenosis, 36
Iodinated contrast material, in
transjugular intrahepatic
portosystemic shunt
placement, complications of,
221

K

Kinks and coils of carotid artery,
77-85
diagnosis, 79
endarterectomy combined with
shortening of internal
carotid for, 81-82
plication of redundant common
carotid in, 83
etiology, 78
incidence, 77-78
signs and symptoms, 78-79
surgery for, 80-83
indications, 79-80
Knee surgery, orthopedic, low-
molecular weight heparin in,
184

L

Laboratory tests, before
portosystemic shunting,
transjugular intrahepatic, 205
Laparoscopy
abdominal aortic aneurysm
repair by, 123-136
clinical experience, 128-132
diet after, clear liquid, interval
to tolerating, 131
future developments, 133-134

hospitalization after, length of,
132
hours to extubation after, 131
ICU stay after, duration of, 132
laparoscopic times in, 130
lessons learned, 132-133
minilaparotomy location in,
127
nasogastric suction after,
duration of, 131
operating room times in, 130
operative technique, 125-128
positions of operative team
members during, 126
trocars in, placement of, 127
use in vascular surgery, 124-125
Lectures, education, in Brown
vascular exercise program
for claudication, 154
Length of stay
after endovascular in situ bypass,
145
after laparoscopic abdominal
aortic aneurysm repair, 132
Lepirudin, 185
in heparin-induced
thrombocytopenia and
thrombosis syndrome,
182-183
Limb (*see* Extremity)
Liver
(*See also* Hepatic)
failure as contraindication to
transjugular intrahepatic
portosystemic shunts, 201
function tests after portosystemic
shunt placement,
transjugular intrahepatic,
218
Lymph node biopsy, laparoscopic
para-aortic, 124

M

Marfan syndrome, propranolol in,
232

Metalloproteinase inhibition, of
aortic aneurysm expansion,
235-237

Metoprolol, inhibition of aortic
aneurysm expansion by, 234

Minilaparotomy, location in
laparoscopic surgery for
abdominal aortic aneurysm,
127

Morbidity
co-morbidity (*see* Co-morbidity)
of heparin-induced
thrombocytopenia and
thrombosis syndrome, 182
perioperative, of carotid
endarterectomy for
asymptomatic patients,
26-28

Mortality
of endovascular abdominal aortic
aneurysm repair, 96
of heparin-induced
thrombocytopenia and
thrombosis syndrome, 182
perioperative, of carotid
endarterectomy for
asymptomatic patients,
26-28
rates in carotid endarterectomy,
3-6

N

NASCET criteria, for duplex
scanning of internal carotid
artery stenosis, 47-48

Nasogastric suction duration, after
laparoscopic abdominal
aortic aneurysm repair, 131

Novastan, in heparin-induced
thrombocytopenia and
thrombosis syndrome, 182

Nursing evaluation, in phase 1 of
Brown vascular exercise
program for claudication,
150-151

O

Occlusion
side branch
in endovascular in situ bypass,
technique, 139-146
Side Branch Occlusion System
in endovascular in situ
bypass, 137-138
stent, after portosystemic shunt
placement, transjugular
intrahepatic, 220
relation to biliary-venous
fistula, 217

Octreotide, discontinuation
after transjugular
intrahepatic portosystemic
shunt, 214

Oculoplethysmography, in
diagnosis of carotid kinks
and coils, 79

Operating
team positions during
laparoscopic surgery for
abdominal aortic aneurysm,
126
times in laparoscopic abdominal
aortic aneurysm repair,
130

Organan, in heparin-induced
thrombocytopenia and
thrombosis syndrome, 182

Orthopedic hip and knee surgery,
low-molecular weight
heparin in, 184

Osteoporosis, after long-term
heparin usage, 182

P

Pain, abdominal, after transjugular
intrahepatic portosystemic
shunt, 213

Patch angioplasty in carotid
endarterectomy
eversion, 57

vs. primary closure (*see*
Endarterectomy, carotid,
closure, primary *vs.* patch
angioplasty)
Patient preparation, before
transjugular intrahepatic
portosystemic shunt,
204-206
Pentoxifylline, for claudication,
160-161
Percutaneous transluminal
angioplasty (*see* Angioplasty,
percutaneous transluminal)
Pericardial disease, restrictive, as
contraindication to
transjugular intrahepatic
portosystemic shunts, 201
Peristomal variceal bleeding,
shunt for (*see* Shunt,
portosystemic, transjugular
intrahepatic)
Persantine, 186
/aspirin, effect on early graft
patency after infrainguinal
revascularization, 168-169
Personnel requirements, for
Brown vascular exercise
program for claudication,
149
Pharmacologic inhibition, of aortic
aneurysm expansion,
229-242
Plaque
carotid, internal, elevation in
eversion endarterectomy, 63
removal and visualization of end
point in eversion carotid
endarterectomy, 64
Polycarbonate, as endovascular
graft material for repair of
abdominal aortic aneurysms,
92
Polyester-covered stents, in
transjugular intrahepatic
portosystemic shunting, 224

Polytetrafluoroethylene (*see* PTFE)
Polyurethane, spun, as
endovascular graft material
for repair of abdominal
aortic aneurysms, 92
Portal vein
access set, Rosch-Uchida system,
206
localization in transjugular
intrahepatic portosystemic
shunting, 206-209
thrombosis
early after transjugular
intrahepatic portosystemic
shunting, 223
portosystemic shunting and,
transjugular intrahepatic,
202
Portography, CO_2 hepatic wedge,
for portal vein localization
for transjugular intrahepatic
portosystemic shunt,
206-208
Portosystemic shunt, transjugular
intrahepatic (*see* Shunt,
portosystemic, transjugular
intrahepatic)
Propranolol
inhibition of aortic aneurysm
expansion
clinical evidence, 232-235
experimental evidence, 231-232
in Marfan syndrome, 232
Prosthesis, sutureless, for aortic
replacement, 134
PTFE
-covered stents in transjugular
intrahepatic portosystemic
shunting, 224
as endovascular graft material for
repair of abdominal aortic
aneurysms, 92
patch *vs.* saphenous vein closure
after carotid endarterectomy,
15-18

Pulmonary
  embolism, low-molecular weight
    heparin in, 184
  hypertension as contraindication
    to transjugular intrahepatic
    portosystemic shunts, 201
Puncture, arterial, during
  transjugular intrahepatic
  portosystemic shunt
  placement, 216

Q

Quality of life measurements, after
  completion of Brown
  exercise program for
  claudication, 157-159

R

Race of asymptomatic patients
  undergoing carotid
  endarterectomy
  death and
    late, 30
    perioperative, 29
  stroke and, perioperative, 28
Radiation-induced skin changes,
  association with transjugular
  intrahepatic portosystemic
  shunts, 221-222
Randomized trials, prospective,
  impact on decision making
  for asymptomatic patients
  with critical carotid stenosis,
  23-24
Reanastomosis
  of internal to common carotid
    artery in eversion
    endarterectomy, 67
  with shunt in place in eversion
    carotid endarterectomy, 69
Refludan, 185
  in heparin-induced
    thrombocytopenia and
    thrombosis syndrome,
    182-183

Reimbursement, for exercise
  program for claudication,
  159-160
Renal failure, association with
  transjugular intrahepatic
  portosystemic shunts, 221
Resources, for Brown vascular
  exercise program for
  claudication, 149-150
Restenosis, carotid artery, after
  endarterectomy
  eversion, after primary closure or
    patch angioplasty, 57
  with greater saphenous vein
    patching *vs.* synthetic
    patching and everted
    cervical vein patching, 17
  with primary closure *vs.* patch
    angioplasty, 13
Revascularization, infrainguinal
  ancrod in, 185
  anticoagulation for (*see*
    Anticoagulation for
    infrainguinal
    revascularization)
Rosch-Uchida system portal vein
  access set, 206

S

Saphenous vein
  bypass, endovascular in situ (*see*
    Bypass, endovascular in
    situ)
  greater, autologous, *vs.* synthetic
    patches in closure after
    carotid endarterectomy, 15-18
Sedation, conscious, transjugular
  intrahepatic portosystemic
  shunting under, 206, 213
Sex
  effect on death after carotid
    endarterectomy for
    asymptomatic patients
    late, 30
    perioperative, 29

effect on perioperative strokes
after carotid endarterectomy
for asymptomatic patients,
28
Shunt
in carotid endarterectomy,
eversion, 68-69
portosystemic, transjugular
intrahepatic, 199-227
complications, 215-222
contraindications, 200-204
future of, 224
indications, 200-204
patency, 222-224
patient preparation before,
204-206
postprocedural care, 212-215
procedural technique, 206-212
results, 215
stent occlusion after, related to
biliary-venous fistula, 217
surveillance after, 222-224
thrombosis early after, 214
Side branch
embolization in endovascular in
situ bypass, 141
occlusion
in endovascular in situ bypass,
technique, 139-146
Side Branch Occlusion System
in endovascular in situ
bypass, 137-138
orifice in endovascular in situ
bypass, angioscopic imaging
of, 140
Skin, changes, radiation-induced,
association with transjugular
intrahepatic portosystemic
shunts, 221-222
Space requirements, for Brown
vascular exercise program
for claudication, 149-150
Spatial orientation, in three-
dimensional ultrasound,
194-195

Spectral analysis, of carotid artery
occlusive disease, 41-53
Splenic artery aneurysm,
laparoscopic ligation of, 124
Stenosis
carotid artery
critical, asymptomatic patients
with, decision making for,
23-39
duplex scanning of (*see*
Ultrasound, duplex, of
carotid artery stenosis)
endarterectomy for (*see*
Endarterectomy, carotid)
delayed, of hepatic vein, after
transjugular intrahepatic
portosystemic shunt
placement, 220
restenosis (*see* Restenosis)
Stent
covered, in transjugular
intrahepatic portosystemic
shunting, 224
occlusion after portosystemic
shunt placement, transjugular
intrahepatic, 220
to vena cava, inferior, in Budd-
Chiari syndrome, 204
Stroke, perioperative, in carotid
endarterectomy, 3-6
in asymptomatic patients, impact
of age, sex, race, and co-
morbidity on, 28
with primary closure *vs.* patch
angioplasty, 12
rate with greater saphenous vein
patching *vs.* synthetic
patching and everted
cervical vein patching, 16
Suction, nasogastric, duration
after laparoscopic abdominal
aortic aneurysm repair, 131
Surgeon
carotid endarterectomy
outcomes, 6-8

case volume, effect on outcome
of carotid endarterectomy in
asymptomatic patients,
34-36
Sutureless prosthesis, for aortic
replacement, 134

T

Talent graft for endovascular
repair of abdominal aortic
aneurysms, 95
attachment system, 91-92
features, 90
Thrombin inhibitors, in heparin-
induced thrombocytopenia
and thrombosis syndrome,
182
Thrombocytopenia and
thrombosis syndrome,
heparin-induced, 182
Thrombosis
early after portosystemic
shunting, transjugular
intrahepatic, 214
thrombocytopenia and
thrombosis syndrome,
heparin-induced, 182
vein
deep, low-molecular weight
heparin in, 184
portal, and transjugular
intrahepatic portosystemic
shunts, 202
portal, early after transjugular
intrahepatic portosystemic
shunting, 223
Tibial in situ bypass, endovascular
femoroposterior
completion arteriogram after, 142
performed through two
incisions, 143
Ticlopidine, 186
effect on graft patency in
infrainguinal
revascularization

early, 169
long-term, 171
Tomography, computed (*see* CT)
Transjugular intrahepatic
portosystemic shunt (*see*
Shunt, portosystemic,
transjugular intrahepatic)
Treadmill test, progressive, before
Brown vascular exercise
program for claudication,
151-153
Trials, prospective randomized,
impact on decision making
for asymptomatic patients
with critical carotid stenosis,
23-24
Trocars, placement in laparoscopic
surgery for abdominal aortic
aneurysm, 127

U

Ultrasound
Doppler
B-mode, real-time in diagnosis
of carotid kinks and coils,
79
color, before portosystemic
shunting, transjugular
intrahepatic, 205
color, for surveillance after
transjugular intrahepatic
portosystemic shunting, 222,
224
energy imaging, color, 191
duplex
of carotid artery occlusive
disease (*see* Ultrasound,
duplex, of carotid stenosis
below)
of carotid artery stenosis, 37
of carotid artery stenosis, in
asymptomatic patients, 37
of carotid artery stenosis,
internal (*see below*)
development, 190-192

three-dimensional *(see*
Ultrasound, three-
dimensional *below)*
duplex, of carotid artery stenosis,
internal, 41-53
bilateral, 50-52
criteria, ACAS, 49-50
criteria, NASCET, 47-48
criteria, supplemental, 46-50
criteria, University of
Washington, 45
for quantification, 42-46
intravascular, in carotid stenosis,
36
three-dimensional, 189-198
flow phantom for, 196
flow phantom for, coronal view,
197
potential applications for,
197-198
spatial orientation and, 194-195
system, development of, 192-194
system, development of,
preliminary development at
Stanford, 196-197
volume visualization, 195-196
University of Washington duplex
criteria, to grade carotid
stenosis, 45

V

Valvulotome, Fogarty, in
endovascular in situ bypass,
137, 138
cutting blade extended,
illustration, 139
Valvulotomy in endovascular in
situ bypass, technique,
138-139
Vanguard graft, for endovascular
repair of abdominal aortic
aneurysms, features of, 90
Variceal bleeding, shunt for *(see*
Shunt, portosystemic,
transjugular intrahepatic)

Vascular
endovascular
bypass, in situ *(see* Bypass,
endovascular in situ)
graft for abdominal aortic
aneurysm repair (see
Endovascular, graft for
abdominal aortic aneurysm
repair)
exercise program *(see* Exercise
program for claudication)
intravascular ultrasound in
carotid stenosis, 36
surgery
carbon dioxide insufflation for,
and air emboli, 133
laparoscopy use in, 124-125
testing, noninvasive, before
Brown vascular exercise
program for claudication,
151
Vein
biliary-venous fistula related to
stent occlusion after
transjugular intrahepatic
portosystemic shunt
placement, 217
cervical, everted, patches, *vs.*
saphenous vein closure after
carotid endarterectomy, 15-18
deep, thrombosis, low-molecular
weight heparin in, 184
hepatic, delayed stenosis, after
transjugular intrahepatic
portosystemic shunt
placement, 220
portal *(see* Portal, vein)
saphenous
bypass, endovascular in situ
(see Bypass, endovascular in
situ)
greater, autologous, *vs.*
synthetic patches in closure
after carotid endarterectomy,
15-18

Vena cava, inferior, Budd-Chiari
   stenting to, 204

W

Walking
   ability after completion of Brown
      vascular exercise program
      for claudication, 155-157
   distance after exercise therapy
      vs. percutaneous
      transluminal angioplasty for
      claudication, 163
Wallstent
   for endoleak, 110
   for limb dysfunction after
      endovascular graft repair of
      abdominal aortic aneurysm,
      100, 101

with portosystemic shunt,
   transjugular intrahepatic,
   210, 212
Warfarin in infrainguinal
   revascularization
with aspirin, 174-176
   effect on long-term graft
      patency, 172
   effect on long-term graft patency,
      172
   long-term usage, 175

Z

Zenith graft, for endovascular
   repair of abdominal aortic
   aneurysms, features of,
   90